AF333601

WORKBOOK TO ACCOMPANY
HUMAN RELATIONS
NOURISHMENT FOR THE MEDICAL PRACTICE

ARLIN V. PETERSON, EdD
ROY C. ALLEN, EdD

Workbook to accompany:
*Human Relations
Nourishment for the Medical Practice*
revised by
Arlin V. Peterson, EdD
Copyright 2003

Originally published as
Human Relations for the Medical Office
by
Arlin V. Peterson, EdD
Roy C. Allen, EdD
Copyright 1978

All rights reserved. American Association of Medical Assistants, Inc. No part of this publication may be reproduced, stored in a retrieval system, or transmitted, in any form or by any means, electronic, mechanical, photocopying, recording, or otherwise, without the prior written permission of the publisher.

ISBN: 0-942732-06-5

Introduction

This workbook is designed to reinforce and supplement your understanding of the concepts presented in *Human Relations: Nourishment for the Medical Practice.* Each chapter in this workbook corresponds to its like-numbered chapter in the book, and the two should be used conjunctively.

You may proceed through this workbook at your own learning pace, since it was intended for use as a self-study aid. The material, however, can be used in study groups, and if you are planning to participate in group study, we suggest that you read the Guidelines for Group Study on page v, as well as the guidelines on the title page of each workbook chapter.

Each chapter commences with a short examination called a "pretest." If you are competent in certain areas of human relations, it may not be necessary for you to study each chapter in the book; to determine your competence, you may "challenge" a chapter by taking the pretest. If you answer the stipulated number of questions correctly, you will have demonstrated your mastery of that material and should proceed directly to the workbook activities. Even if you feel you cannot successfully challenge a chapter, reading and attempting to answer the pretest questions will help orient you to the material and heighten your awareness of the key concepts when you study the chapter.

Also to be found in each of the workbook chapters are "Personal Practice Learning Activities," exercises designed to:

1. Provide an opportunity for you to explore your personal and professional life.
2. Facilitate your awareness of self and others, as well as your interactions.
3. Assist you in understanding the influence of your environment on your life.
4. Personalize your learning.

Another examination, referred to as the "posttest," is the concluding element of each chapter, and is to be completed after the chapter has been read and the activities finished. It will measure how well you have mastered the content of the chapter.

A final examination, Form A and Form B, is also included in the workbook, along with a special answer sheet for each form. The completed answer sheet of one form showing that you answered 70 percent of the questions correctly on your first attempt will serve as your evidence to the American Association of Medical Assistants that you have satisfactorily completed its guided study course in human relations and are entitled to 45 CEUs (30 gen, 15 adm) awarded by the AAMA. More complete directions regarding the examination are included in that section of the workbook.

The Personal Practice Learning Activities are the results of the authors' educational and teaching experiences. They are original in the sense that they have been prepared especially for this workbook. However, the original exercises, from which some of these activities have been modified, were developed by many individuals and shared through word of mouth, workshop activities, lecture notes, and mimeographed sheets of unknown authorship. We would like to recognize especially the contributions made by the counselor educators and group facilitators who have been a part of the human growth movement. Special recognition and acknowledgment are given Sidney Simon, EdD, Thomas Gordon, PhD; William Glasser, MD; Carl Rogers, PhD; Robert Carkhuff, PhD; and George Gazda, EdD, for their tremendous contributions to the human relations training movement. Medical assistants using these activities for personal growth or teaching purposes should feel free to use or modify the activities in any manner that satisfies their needs.

Arlin V. Peterson, EdD
Roy C. Allen, EdD

Guidelines for Group Study

This guide is designed to enhance the student's exploration, understanding, and utilization of the materials presented in the book and workbook, *Human Relations Nourishment for the Medical Practice.* It was prepared to aid individuals who wish to *supplement* their independent study with group study. Group study must not replace independent study, but group discussion and sharing are usually very enriching for all individuals, especially when the subject being discussed is human relations.

General guidelines are offered below that apply to every chapter of the materials and every meeting. At the beginning of each chapter in the workbook, specific guidelines for that chapter are presented.

General guidelines

1. The discussions and learning will proceed more effectively and culminate in greater benefit to group members if one member accepts responsibility for leading the discussion. The discussion leader should not attempt to "teach" the material; rather, her responsibilities should include initiating the discussions, encouraging participation from all members, keeping the discussions proceeding and summarizing key points at the conclusion of each meeting. One person may serve as discussion leader for the entire course, or the responsibility may rotate among the group members on a meeting-by-meeting or chapter-by-chapter basis.
2. For general discussions of the book material, the group may be as large as 15 to 20 people. To discuss or conduct the workbook activities, the larger group should be subdivided into smaller groups of approximately six people.
3. The chapter or section of the book and workbook to be discussed should be assigned and read by participants prior to the group meeting.

Where applicable, the personal practice learning activities should also be completed prior to the meeting during which they will be discussed. The pretests should be considered a part of each participant's independent study. Since the pretest questions are identical to the competency check questions, which will be covered during class, meeting time should not be devoted to the pre-test per se.

4. The length of each meeting will depend on the size of the group, the topic(s) being discussed, and the group's interest in the topic(s). As a guide for initial planning, however, we suggest that two hours be set aside for each meeting according to the following schedule:

   A. 45 minutes to discuss the material in the book.
   B. 45 minutes to discuss and, where applicable, do the personal practice learning activities. More specific direction is included in the chapter guidelines.
   C. 15 minutes to discuss post-test questions. We recommend that group members answer and score their own post-tests outside of class, but that a small portion of class time be devoted to discussing any troublesome or difficult questions.
   D. 15 minutes to discuss related reading and miscellaneous, but relevant, topics of group interest.

5. Usually each chapter in the book and its corresponding chapter in the workbook will provide sufficient material for one two-hour discussion, but if the group prefers to proceed more slowly, each chapter can be broken into subunits of study according to the topics covered in each. More specific direction is included in the chapter guidelines.
6. General topics for discussion during each session include:

A. A comment from each group member regarding what she felt were the most important and useful ideas from the assigned reading.

B. The competency check questions and chapter objectives.

C. Key concepts not covered in the competency checks.

D. How to apply the concepts presented to one's job setting and personal life.

E. Those personal practice learning activities of most interest to the group. Most of the assigned learning activities should be completed prior to class, with class time devoted to discussing them. However, group members should not be forced to participate in any activity which is threatening to them ... members should share only material they feel comfortable about sharing.

F. Identifying problems common to group members and their solutions.

G. A statement from each group member regarding what she has learned of personal value or an idea she will try to implement.

7. The final examination is designed for individual use, but it may be administered in a group setting if this is preferred. If so, and additional two-hour meeting should be scheduled for its administration.

Most people will probably be able to complete the examination in approximately one hour, but no one should be rushed to do so. After everyone has completed her examination, the group may wish to utilize remaining time in discussing the questions.

Each group member can send her examination response sheet to AAMA headquarters herself, but it would be more efficient if the discussion leader collected them at the end of the meeting and forwarded them to AAMA headquarters in bulk.

Table of contents

Chapter 1:

Why study human relations?

Guidelines for Group Study   Be sure to read and use the General Guidelines for Group Study in addition to the following Chapter Guidelines.

---

1. From the book:

    A. Review the chapter objectives and competency check question.
    B. Discuss the need to study human relations.
    C. Discuss the facets of social learning theory.

2. From the workbook:

    A. All Personal Practice Learning Activities are appropriate for group discussion.
    B. The activities are arranged in the most beneficial sequence but can be rearranged and discussed in any order.
    C. If the group does not wish to discuss all the activities, Activities 1 and 4 should be given priority in the group setting.

Pretest　　　　In the space provided answer concisely each of the following questions. The answer key follows the pretest.

1.　Define human relations.

2.　Describe a well-adjusted medical assistant.

3.　What is the basic ingredient of personality?

4.　Give the major reason people lose their jobs.

5.　Treating the patient's physical needs is not necessarily effective health care. What other needs must be treated?

6.　Where does human relations improvement begin?

7.　Define social learning.

Pretest

8. Briefly distinguish between socialization and individualization.

9. Explain how social factors can play an important role in shaping emotional behavior.

10. Define the terms "identification" and "imitation" as they relate to a person's behavior.

11. How does socially acceptable behavior relate to self-concept?

12. Applying appropriate principles of social learning theory, describe how the medical assistant can influence the reactions of waiting patients to the announcement that the physician will be late in getting to the office.

Pretest
Answer Key

Compare your responses to the pretest questions to the correct answers stated in the following key. If you answer nine of the twelve questions correctly, proceed to the Personal Practice Learning Activities, as you have successfully challenged the content of this chapter. If fewer than nine of your answers are correct, you should study the material in Chapter I of the book.

Your answers need not correspond exactly to the answers in the key below, but the meanings of the two responses must be similar in order for your answer to be considered correct.

---

1. Human relations is the science of dealing with people in such a way that our self-image and their self-image remain positive and intact.

2. A well-adjusted medical assistant enjoys people from all walks of life and has the ability to deal with them effectively.

3. The basic ingredient of personality is the ability to get along with other people.

4. The major reason people lose their jobs is that they have not developed the personalities needed for successfully dealing with other people.

5. In addition to providing treatment for illness, the emotional and psychological needs of the patient must be treated.

6. Improving human relations must begin with ourselves.

7. Social learning is the acquisition of the behavioral patterns expected by society.

8. Society's attempt to have us accept its regulations, values, and morals may be described as socialization; individualization refers to our attempts to retain our own individuality, while at the same time making certain compromises or concessions to obtain group acceptance.

9. The better our social life, the healthier our mental condition will be. Our emotional behavior is influenced by the social environment in which we live and work.

10. If a person assumes the roles, attitudes, feelings, and behavior of another person, the principle of identification is practiced. Imitation refers to the principle of copying another person's behavior.

11. Socially acceptable behavior is essentially a matter of developing a self-concept in which one's needs and purposes are integrated with those of the social group for the mutual benefit of both.

12. The patients' reaction to this announcement will likely be taken from the attitude of the medical assistant. If the medical assistant maintains a happy, friendly atmosphere and smiles and talks with the patients, they are less likely to be upset by the lateness of the physician.

Personal Practice Learning Activities

The following activities are designed to provide you with an opportunity to explore your personal and professional lives. Many of you have probably not taken the time to examine where you have been, where you are now, or where you are going. If you don't determine where you want to go, you may not get there; if you do not plan your route, you may end up somewhere else.

1. Your personal lifeline

    A. The line below is your personal lifeline. The dot on the far left is you birthdate. The dot on the far right is your anticipated death year. Write in those years.

    B. Place a dot that indicates your present position on your lifeline. Put today's date by your dot.

    C. To the left of your present position, list all of your past achievements and happy memories.

    D. To the right of your present position, list all of those things you hope to do or accomplish before your death.

    E. Study and reflect on your lifeline.

    F. Answer the following questions:

        1) I learned that I

        2) I am pleased that I

        3) I hope that I

**Personal Practice
Learning Activities**

---

2. Your professional (medical assistant) lifeline

   A. The line below is your professional lifeline. The dot on the extreme left is the day you became or hope to become a medical assistant. The dot on the far right is your anticipated retirement date. Write in those dates.

   B. Place a dot that indicates your present position on your professional lifeline. Put today's date by your dot.

   C. To the left of your present position, list all of your past achievements and happy memories.

   D. To the right of your present position, list all of those things you hope to do or accomplish before your retirement.

   E. List those things you would like to accomplish after you retire.

   F. Study and reflect on your professional lifeline.

   G. Answer the following questions:

       1) I learned that I

       2) I am pleased that I

       3) I hope that I

**Personal Practice
Learning Activities**

---

3. Inventory of human relations skills

    Consider your relationships with others. You will usually be more or less described as the following sentences indicate. Rate yourself from 1 to 5 according to the following scale: 1, never; 2, seldom; 3, sometimes; 4, usually; or 5, always.

	Never	Seldom	Sometimes	Usually	Always
1. I am considerate.	1	2	3	4	5
2. I am understanding.	1	2	3	4	5
3. I am confident.	1	2	3	4	5
4. I am cheerful.	1	2	3	4	5
5. I am dignified.	1	2	3	4	5
6. I am gracious.	1	2	3	4	5
7. I am agreeable.	1	2	3	4	5
8. I am enthusiastic.	1	2	3	4	5
9. I am calm.	1	2	3	4	5
10. I am quiet.	1	2	3	4	5
11. I am radiant.	1	2	3	4	5
12. I am outgoing.	1	2	3	4	5
13. I am sweet.	1	2	3	4	5
14. I am patient.	1	2	3	4	5
15. I am mature.	1	2	3	4	5
16. I like most people.	1	2	3	4	5
17. I assume others will like me.	1	2	3	4	5
18. I am careful about my appearance.	1	2	3	4	5
19. Most people cooperate with me.	1	2	3	4	5
20. I listen carefully to what others have to say.	1	2	3	4	5
21. I always give others credit for what they do.	1	2	3	4	5
22. I am never impatient in dealing with others.	1	2	3	4	5
23. My temper never gets me in trouble.	1	2	3	4	5
24. I never brag.	1	2	3	4	5
25. I never snub or ignore anyone.	1	2	3	4	5
26. I follow directions well.	1	2	3	4	5
27. I do what needs to be done without being told.	1	2	3	4	5
28. I am a good organizer.	1	2	3	4	5
29. I have good communication skills.	1	2	3	4	5
30. I am happy with me.	1	2	3	4	5

**Personal Practice
Learning Activities**

---

4. Purpose of life

    Answer the following questions:

    A. What is your purpose for living?

    B. What purpose do you serve in being a medical assistant?

    C. How can you make the world a little better place as a result of your having lived?

    D. How would you like to be described as a person upon your death?

5. Personal objectives
    A. What do you want to happen to you as a result of studying the Human Relations Course?

    B. Describe what you do that justifies your rating yourself as you did on each item in Activity 3.

        1)

        2)

        3)

**Personal Practice
Learning Activities**

---

4)

5)

6)

7)

8)

9)

10)

11)

12)

13)

14)

**Personal Practice
Learning Activities**

---

15)

16)

17)

18)

19)

20)

21)

22)

23)

24)

25)

**Personal Practice
Learning Activities**

---

26)

27)

28)

29)

30)

C.   From these 30 items list the three things you frequently do that please you the most.

D.   From these 30 items list the three things you least like about yourself.

E.   List those areas of your personal life that you would like to be able to improve.

Post-Test As concisely as possible, answer each of the following questions without referring to your book or other material. When finished, refer to the Chapter I post-test answer key.

1. Briefly describe interpersonal relationship skills and their function.

2. Define human relations.

3. Explain how an irritating interaction away from your job will influence your satisfaction and efficiency.

4. What is the relationship between social learning and social behavior?

5. The medical assistant's behavior relates to the social expectations of her role. Give an example.

6. Explain how a socially skilled medical assistant might have the opportunity to further develop her social skills.

7. Much human learning is the result of observing the behavior of others. Explain how this statement relates to social learning.

Post-Test

8. What do most authorities believe to be the single most important characteristic distinguishing between effective and ineffective personnel?

9. What is a necessary condition for the development of social control?

10. List two types of reinforcement with an example of each.

11. How does socially acceptable behavior relate to self-concept?

12. How is social and emotional maturity best promoted?

**Post-Test
Answer Key**

Compare your answers to the post-test questions to the correct answers given in the following key. While your response to each question need not correspond exactly with the words used in the answers below, the meanings must be similar in order for your response to be considered correct.

If you answer nine of the twelve questions correctly, you have demonstrated a satisfactory understanding of the material in Chapter I and should proceed to the Personal Practice Learning Activities if you have not completed them or to Chapter II if you have. If you answer fewer that nine questions correctly, you should restudy the appropriate sections of Chapter I before proceeding.

---

1. Interpersonal relationship skills are the personal skills we develop which enable us to get along with other people in a way that will bring personal satisfaction but not degrade or hinder our self-concept, self-image, and ego or the self-concept, self-image, and ego of those with whom we deal.

2. Human relations is the science of dealing with people in such a way that our self-image and their self-image remain positive and intact.

3. Interactions away from the job influence our mood or attitude on the job. For example, a conflict with our spouse before work cannot help but hinder our attitude, awareness, and efficiency on the job.

4. As situations change from one environment to another, we first learn and then demonstrate the socially expected and accepted behavior of the new environment.

5. Society expects responsible social behavior from members of responsible professions. For example, a medical assistant has knowledge of very personal information about the patient. Socially, as well as ethically, the medical assistant is expected to keep this information confidential.

6. A socially skilled person receives more social invitations and, therefore, has more opportunities to further develop and improve her social skills.

7. Much social learning is accomplished by identifying with and imitating those significant others in our lives who are socially accepted.

8. The interpersonal relationship skills which have or have not been developed are the most important characteristic.

9. Learning that other people are important is a necessary condition for the development of social control.

10. External reinforcement, such as a paycheck, and internal reinforcement, such as self-satisfaction, are two types.

Post-Test Answer Key

---

11. Socially acceptable behavior is essentially a matter of developing a self-concept in which one's needs and purposes are integrated with those of thc social group for the mutual benefit of both.

12. Social and emotional maturity are best promoted through the dual process of creating a secure environment and the opportunity to practice socially productive behavior.

Related readings

---

1. Aspy D. *Toward a Technology for Humanizing Education.* Champaign, Ill: Research Press Co; 1972.

2. Gazda G, Walters R, Childers W. *Human Relations Development, A Manual of Health Sciences.* Boston, Mass: Allyn & Bacon Inc; 1975.

3. Giblin L. *How to Have Confidence and Power in Dealing with People.* Englewood Cliffs, NJ: Prentice-Hall Inc; 1956.

4. Glasser W. *Mental Health or Mental Illness.* New York, NY: Harper & Row; 1970.

5. Glasser W. *Schools Without Failure.* New York, NY: Harper & Row; 1969.

6. Lair J. *I Ain't Much Baby, But I'm All I've Got.* Garden City, NY: Doubleday & Co; 1969.

7. May R. *Man's Search for Himself.* New York, NY: Delta Publishing Co; 1953.

Additional Readings

Canfield J, Hanson M. *Chicken Soup for the Soul.* Deerfield Beach, Fla: Health Communications Inc; 1993.

Carlson R. *Don't Sweat the Small Stuff and It's All Small Stuff.* New York, NY: Hyperion; 1997.

Kushner H. *When All You've Ever Wanted Isn't Enough.* New York, NY: Pocket Book; 1986.

Peck M. *Further Along the Road Less Traveled.* New York, NY: Simon and Schuster; 1993.

Peck M. *The Road Less Traveled and Beyond.* New York, NY: Simon and Schuster; 1997.

Robbins A. *Unlimited Power.* New York, NY: Ballantine Books; 1986.

Chapter II:

Understanding human behavior

<table>
<tr><td>Guidelines for
Group Study</td><td>Because of the many theories and concept presented in Chapter II, the group may wish to devote two class sessions to it.</td></tr>
</table>

1. From the book:

   A. Discuss the chapter objectives and competency check questions.
   B. Discuss the following theories or concepts:
      1) The causal approach to understanding human behavior.
      2) Maslow's Hierarchy of Needs.
      3) Perceptual psychology.
      4) Effectiveness training.
      5) Transactional analysis.
      6) Choice Theory
      7) Seven Habits

2. From the workbook:

   A. Activities 1, 2, 3, and 5 are appropriate for group discussion. Each member should share her responses to these activities.
   B. Activity 4 can be discussed, or the group may prefer to simulate and role-play the conversations requested.
   C. If time is limited, Activities 1 and 4 should be given priority during the meeting.

Pretest   In the space provided answer concisely each of the following questions. The answer key follows the pretest.

---

1. How do an individual's interactions with other people affect an individual's private behavior?

2. Explain the Behavior Equation: MF + R + IPS = Behavior.

3. Describe how the Behavior Equation may be used to understand your own behavior and the behavior of other medical assistants in your office.

4. List Maslow's hierarchy of needs. How do the five levels interrelate?

5. Explain why a medical assistant who has reached a higher degree of self-actualization is likely to be more productive than a medical assistant who has achieved a lesser degree of self-actualization.

6. How do Glasser's basic needs of love, belonging and power correspond to Maslow's hierarchy of needs?

7. Differentiate between perceptual psychology and the causal approach.

Pretest

---

8. According to perceptual psychologists, what determines how an individual behaves in a particular situation?

9. How do our attitudes about ourselves affect our acceptance of others?

10. Explain Gordon's concept of problem ownership.

11. Briefly explain Transactional Analysis.

12. List and define the three ego states.

13. According to the TA model, explain why strokes are essential.

14. Differentiate between the positions, "I'm not OK, you're OK" and "I'm OK, you're OK" as they apply to daily living.

15. List the four psychological needs presented in Choice Theory.

16. What are the four components of total behavior?

17. Explain Covey's notion of synergize.

18. What does it mean to sharpen the saw?

**Pretest
Answer Key**

Compare your pretest responses to the correct answers stated in the following key. If you answer eleven of the fourteen questions correctly, proceed to the Personal Practice Learning Activities, as you have successfully challenged the content of the chapter. If fewer then eleven of your answers are correct, then you should study the material in Chapter II of the book.

Your answers need not correspond exactly to the answers in the key, but the meaning of the two responses must be similar in order for your answer to be considered correct.

---

1. An individual's interactions with other people determine to a great extent whether his own wants and needs are satisfied and whether he is a happy, healthy, contented person.

2. MF: Motivating Force(s) of individual needs, i.e., the need for self-respect.
   R. Personal Resources, i.e., skills, talents, capabilities.
   IPS: Immediate Physical Setting, i.e, the time and place in which the behavior occurs.

3. The secret to utilizing the Behavior Equation, to understanding your own behavior or the behavior of others, is to look at and attempt to identify the various factors that are interacting.

4. There are five levels in Maslow's hierarchy of needs. The first is the need for survival, i.e., the need for food and shelter. Physical safety or freedom from personal harm is the second basic need. Maslow defines the third basic need as the need for love and a sense of belonging, such as obtaining mutual trust, understanding, and acceptance. The fourth basic need is the need to feel of value and worth, the need for self-respect and the respect of others. The fifth and last basic need is for self-actualization and the opportunity to function to our maximum potential and grow as a person. Each of the five basic needs relate to another in that the prior need must be satisfied before the succeeding need can be met.

5. A self-actualized medical assistant has achieved a sense of purpose and meaning in her life. Therefore, she is not concerned with herself and has the capacity to think of mankind.

6. Glasser's need to love and to be loved corresponds with Maslow's third level needs, the need for love and a sense of belonging. Glasser's need for power corresponds with Maslow's fourth level needs, which he calls the "esteem needs."

7. Perceptual psychologists attempt to understand behavior from the person's viewpoint while proponents of the causal approach consider behavior the result of outside forces influencing the individual.

8. A person's perception of herself and others combined with her perceptions of her immediate world environment will determine how she behaves.

9. When satisfied with our physical and emotional self, we are more accepting of others.

Pretest Answer Key

10. Gordon's concept of problem ownership states that the person experiencing unacceptable behavior is the person who owns the problem. For example, if I do not approve of your behavior, it is my problem, not yours.

11. Transactional Analysis suggests that behavior can be understood by considering transactions between various ego states. The ego states are parent, adult, and child.

12. The parent ego state is simply those things we have taken in and recorded our "tape" from our parents. The adult ego state is viewed as a human computer which stores the information fed it and retrieves this information for decisions that have to be made. The child ego state is said to be our carefree, spontaneous, and emotional state.

13. According to the TA model, strokes, whether positive or negative, are essential because they are basically recognition.

14. The OK Theory basically demonstrates how we feel about ourselves. The position "I'm not OK, you're OK" indicates you value the other person more than yourself. The "I'm OK, you're OK" position presents both individuals on the same emotional link.

15. Love and belonging, power, freedom, and fun.

16. Doing, thinking, feeling, physiology.

17. According to Covey, synergize is the process of finding a third alternative way that is better than what any one individual might propose.

18. Seek opportunities for continuous growth and development.

**Personal Practice
Learning Activities**

Some behavior we like, some behavior we do not. Sometimes we do things we are proud of, and sometimes we do things of which we are not so proud. The following activities are designed to help you become more aware of the reasons for certain behaviors and your reactions to them.

1. Behavior assessment

    A. List on the left the kinds of behavior you appreciate from you friends, and on the right behaviors you do <u>not</u> appreciate.

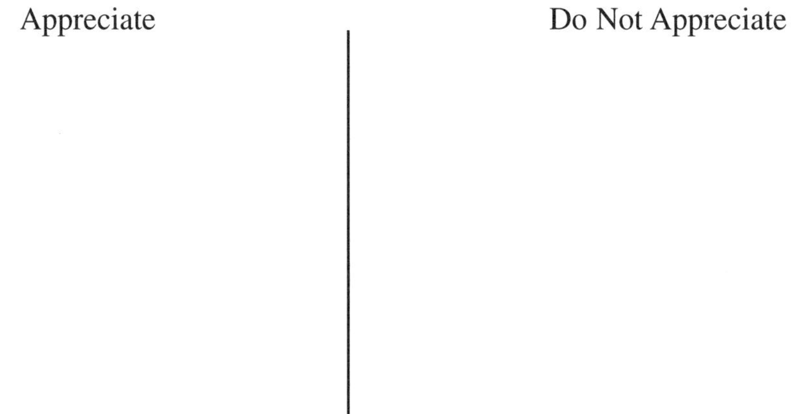

    B. List on the left the kinds of behavior that you appreciate from your boss, and on the right behaviors that you do <u>not</u> appreciate.

Appreciate   Do Not Appreciate

Personal Practice
Learning Activities

C. List on the left the kinds of behavior that you appreciate from your co-workers, and on the right the behaviors you do <u>not</u> appreciate.

Appreciate | Do not Appreciate

D. List on the left the kinds of behavior you exhibit that your friends, boss, and co-workers appreciate, and on the right the behaviors they do <u>not</u> appreciate.

Appreciate | Do not Appreciate

2. Assessing job behavior

A. Why do you work?

**Personal Practice
Learning Activities**

B. List acceptable job behaviors.

C. List unacceptable job behaviors.

D. How does your local community affect your job behavior?

E. How do your office size, location, and physical facilities affect your job behavior?

F. How does your job behavior carry over to your personal life?

3. Dreaming

Describe the perfect medical assistant and the ideal job situation.

Personal Practice
Learning Activities

---

4. Talking

    A. Imagine a conversation with your boss and tell him everything you have thought but never said to him or her. (Write your conversation.) How would your boss answer you?

    B. Be your boss and tell yourself to shape up or what to do. (Write your conversation.) How would you respond?

    C. Think of the worst patient with whom you have ever had contact and tell him/her what you think of him/her. (Write your conversation.) How would he/she respond?

**Personal Practice
Learning Activities**

D. Think of the best patient with whom you have ever had contact and tell him/her what you think of him/her. (Write your conversation.) How would he/she respond?

E. Have your "parent" talk to your "child." How would your child respond?

F. Have your "adult" talk to your "parent." How would your parent respond?

**Personal Practice
Learning Activities**

G. Discuss with yourself what you have learned about human behavior. (Write your conclusions.)

5. Ego states and feelings

A. What behavior have you copied from your mother?

B. What behavior have you copied from your father?

C. Think and write one parental message you still hear in your head that you either obey, resist, or about which you feel confused.

D. Think and write about a recent decision you made after gathering the data and facts needed to make the best possible decision. Contrast this "adult" decision with another decision you made from your "child" ego state.

**Personal Practice
Learning Activities**

E. Imagine you have gone to work as usual. Your boss is there to meet you, and he/she is tense, angry, and jumps on you for something you forgot to do.

1) What are your feelings or thoughts?

2) What would you do?

3) How did you respond to your parents or teachers as a child in similar situations?

4) What would your parents do?

5) How do you feel now?

6) What do you think is the best thing to do about the situation with your boss?

PETE'S PATHOGRAM

9													
			X X		X X		X X		X X		X X		X X
8			X X		X X		X X		X X		X X		X X
7	⊕		X X		X X		X X		X X		X X		X X
6			X X		X X		X X		X X		X X		X X
5	○		X X		X X		X X		X X		X X		X X
4		○	X X		X X		X X		X X		X X		X X
3			X X		X X		X X		X X		X X		X X
2			X X		X X		X X		X X		X X		X X
1			X X		X X		X X		X X		X X		X X
	***SAMPLE**		**BELONGING** Loving Cooperating		**POWER** Competing Achieving		**FREEDOM** Moving Choosing		**FUN** Learning Playing		**SURVIVAL** Risking Reproducing	

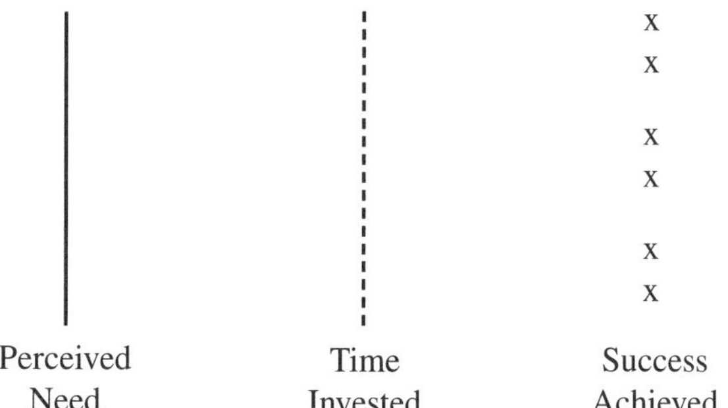

*Plot by circling the appropriate number—Perceived need, time invested and success achieved for all five genetic needs.

Pete's Pathogram
Instruction

---

1. Determine which of the five basic needs seems to be of most importance to you at the present time. On a scale of 1-9, plot the intensity of the need as illustrated on Pete's Pathogram. This will be your highest need line.

2. Determine which of the five basic needs seems to have the least importance to you at the present time. On a scale of 1-9, plot the intensity of that need as illustrated on Pete's Pathogram. This will be your shortest need line.

3. On a scale of 1-9, plot the intensity of your need for the remaining three basic needs. These lines will be between your highest and lowest perceived need lines.

4. Use the same procedure to plot the five lines on the 1-9 scale for the amount of time you invest in attempting to satisfy each need. Plot as illustrated on Pete's Pathogram. These lines may or may not be the same as your perceived need lines.

5. Use the same procedure to plot the five lines on the 1-9 scale for the success you are having in satisfying each of your basic needs. Plot as illustrated on Pete's Pathograms. The success line may or may not be the same as perceived need or time invested lines.

Process guidelines

Study your profile. Do you have appropriate balance or is there a specific reason for the profile to be skewed? Are you spending adequate time trying to satisfy the needs most important to you? Are you having success in proportion to time and energy spent? In other words, is what you're doing working or are you having a lot of success without much effort? Maybe you have a real talent that could be used to enhance your psychological strength. Generally, what did you learn about yourself?

Post-Test   As concisely as possible, answer each of the following questions without referring to your textbook or other material. When finished, refer to the Chapter II post-test answer key.

1. How do an individual's interactions with other people affect an individual's private behavior?

2. In the following scenario, identify Medical Assistant B's Motivating Force, Personal Resources, and Immediate Physical Setting.

   In front of the physician-employer and several patients, Medical Assistant A tells Medical Assistant B that she is tactless and needs to study human relations. Medical Assistant B immediately responds with the suggestion that Medical Assistant A "practice what she preaches."

3. According to Maslow, do needs vary among people of different cultures? Do ways for meeting needs vary?

4. Arrange the following needs according to the hierarchy proposed by Maslow: The need to have a meaningful career; the need for food; the need for respect from colleagues; the need to be safe; and the need to express love for another human being.

5. How would perceptual psychologists explain why two people viewing the same event could see and respond differently to it?

Post-Test

---

6. Differentiate between perceptual psychology and the causal approach.

7. Explain how the work environment affects behavior on the job.

8. According to proponents of effectiveness training, what factors cause our emotional line to fluctuate?

9. Giving an example, relate the theory of ownership of problems to a conflict between two medical assistants.

10. Briefly explain Transactional Analysis.

11. List and describe the three child-type ego states.

12. Differentiate between the positions, "I'm not OK, you're OK" and "I'm OK, you're OK" as they relate to daily living.

13. Where, according to Choice Theory, do we store the pictures of the people, places and things that help us meet our basic needs?

14. What is the core question in the Reality Therapy process?

15. List the first three habits suggested by Covey as habits for highly effective people.

<table>
<tr><td>

**Post-Test
Answer Key**

</td><td>

Compare your answers to the post-test questions to the correct answers given in the following key. While your response to each question need not correspond exactly to the words used in the answers below, the meaning must be similar in order for your response to be considered correct.

If you answer nine of the twelve questions correctly, you will have demonstrated a satisfactory understanding of the material in Chapter II and should proceed to the Personal Practice Learning Activities if you have not completed them or to Chapter III if you have. If you answer fewer than nine questions correctly, you should restudy the appropriate sections of Chapter II before proceeding.

</td></tr>
</table>

1. An individual's interactions with other people determine to a great extent whether his own wants and needs are satisfied and whether he is a happy, healthy, contented person.

2. Medical Assistant B's primary Motivating Force (MF) was the need for esteem and respect; her Personal Resources (R) included the abilities to think and retort quickly; and the Immediate Physical Setting (IPS) was, of course, the busy medical office. (While Medical Assistant B's response may have been effective in some respects, it probably did little to enhance communications and the relationship between the two medical assistants.)

3. Maslow states that the basic needs of all cultures are the same but that the ways of meeting those needs vary greatly.

4. Level 1: The need for food
   Level 2: The need to be safe.
   Level 3: The need to express love for another human being.
   Level 4: The need for respect from colleagues.
   Level 5: The need to have a meaningful career.

5. Perceptual psychologists believe that people perceive things according to their emotional state at the moment of the perception. Therefore, two people in different emotional states could see and respond to the same event differently.

6. Perceptual psychologists attempt to understand behavior from the person's viewpoint while proponents of the causal approach consider behavior the result of outside forces influencing the individual.

7. Pleasant surroundings and desirable working conditions set a climate in which we can deal with conflicts more effectively.

8. According to proponents of effectiveness training, the following three factors cause our emotional line to fluctuate: 1) the effects of significant others in our daily lives; 2) the immediate environment; and 3) how we feel about ourselves at any particular moment.

Post-Test Answer Key

---

9. In an office, Medical Assistant A feels that Medical Assistant B is not doing her share of the office work. The physician-employer is not concerned about the situation one way or the other. Therefore, the owner of the problem is Medical Assistant A. (The example in your answer need not be the same, but the same idea must be expressed in order for your answer to be considered correct.)

10. Transactional Analysis suggests that behavior can be understood by considering transactions between various ego states. The ego states are parent, adult, and child.

11. The three types of child ego states are: The adopted child, who is the product of parent training and personal experiences; the little professor, who is emerging and becoming an adult; and the natural child, who is the untrained infant.

12. The "I'm not OK, you're OK" position indicates that you value the other person more than yourself. The "I'm OK, you're OK" position presents both individuals on the same emotional link.

13. Quality World

14. Is what you're doing helping you or getting you what you want?

15. Be proactive, begin with the end in mind, and put first things first.

Related readings

---

1. Berne E. *Games People Play.* New York, NY: Random House; 1964.

2. Calden G. *I Count, You Count.* Chicago, Ill: Argus Communications; 1976.

3. Combs A, Avila D, Purkey W. *Helping Relationships—Basic Concepts for the Helping Professions.* Boston, Mass: Allyn-Bacon Inc; 1971.

4. Ernst K. *Games Students Play.* Millbrae, Calif: Celestial Arts; 1972.

5. Glasser W. *Reality Therapy.* New York, NY: Harper & Row Publishers; 1965.

6. Gordon T. *Parent Effectiveness Training.* New York, NY: Peter H. Wyden Inc; 1970.

7. James M, Jongeward D. *Born to Win.* Redding, Mass: Addleson Wesley Publishing Co; 1971.

8. Harris T. *I'm OK, You're OK. New York,* NY: Harper & Row Publishers; 1967.

9. Steiner C. *Games Alcoholics Play.* New York, NY: Grove Press Inc; 1971.

Additional Readings 35

Glasser W and C. *What Is This Thing Called Love?* Chatsworth, Calif: William Glasser Institute; 2000.

Glasser W. *Staying Together.* New York, NY: Harper Collins; 1995.

Glasser W. *Reality Therapy In Action.* New York, NY: Harper Collins; 2000.

Covey S. *Daily Reflections for Highly Effective People.* New York, NY: Simon and Schuster; 1994.

Covey S. *Living the 7 Habits.* New York, NY: Simon and Schuster; 1999.

Covey S. *Principle-Centered Leadership.* New York, NY: Simon and Schuster; 1991.

Chapter III:

Understanding self and others

Guidelines for Group Study

Because of the length of this chapter, the group may wish to devote two class sessions to it. Remember to allow time to discuss related readings and troublesome Post-Test questions.

---

1. From the book:

    A. Discuss the chapter objectives and competency check questions.
    B. Discuss each of the following:
        1) The importance of self-concept.
        2) Individual strengths and weaknesses.
        3) The physical, psychological, mental and social characteristics of the successful medical assistant.
        4) The importance of the awareness of others.

2. From the workbook:

    A. Activity 1 can be done during class.
    B. Activity 2 can be done during class in pairs. After each pair has completed the first ten statements, small groups should be formed to discuss the last five statements.
    C. Activities 3 and 4 should be completed prior to the group meeting, with the results discussed during class.
    D. Activity 5 can be done during class, and small groups formed to discuss the results.
    E. If time is limited. Activities 1, 4, and 5 should be given priority.

Pretest   In the space provided answer concisely each of the following questions. The answer key follows the pretest.

---

1. State the meaning of "self-concept."

2. Explain the meaning of "feedback" as it relates to building self-concept.

3. One of the most influential factors affecting behavior is:

4. List four ways to promote your self-concept.

5. Differentiate between hereditary and environmental characteristics.

6. How can a person minimize her weakness?

7. In addition to adequate knowledge and technical skill, what is an essential ingredient for being a successful medical assistant?

---

8. List positive self-image characteristics of the successful medical assistant.

9. Explain the desirable relationship between office procedures and patient care.

10. Briefly discuss the importance of a medical assistant's physical appearance.

11. Describe the mental characteristics of a successful medical assistant.

12. Explain the effect a smile has on other people.

13. What are the characteristics of a good conversationalist?

14. To a patient, what may be the most important words in the English language?

15. List and briefly describe the five stages of dying as classified by Elisabeth Kübler-Ross, MD.

Pretest

---

16. Explaining the concept of reciprocal influence.

17. Briefly discuss how to use effective communication when criticism is necessary.

Pretest
Answer Key

Compare your pretest responses to the correct answers stated in the following key. If you answer thirteen of the seventeen questions correctly, proceed to the Personal Practice Learning Activities, as you have successfully challenged the content of this chapter. If fewer than thirteen of your answers are correct, you should study the material in Chapter III of the book.

Your answers need not correspond exactly to the answers in the key, but the meaning of the two responses must be similar in order for your answer to be considered correct.

---

1. Self-concept is the beliefs and attitudes one has about oneself or, in other words, how a person sees himself or herself.

2. Feedback is the reaction a person receives from another as a result of certain behavior. Positive reactions to behavior improve a person's self-concept while negative reactions damage one's self-concept.

3. Self-concept.

4. Self-concept can be promoted by:
    A. Being open and honest with yourself and others.
    B. Speaking and operating from the positive.
    C. Practicing positive communication skills.
    D. Developing an "I'm OK" attitude.

5. Hereditary characteristics are genetic attributes inherited from parents such as physical characteristics and, to some extent, intellectual capacity. Environmental characteristics are those attributes acquired through interactions with others such as teachers, co-workers, and peer group members.

6. A person can minimize her weakness by concentrating on her strengths and those things she does well, by accepting weakness as a challenge rather than an obstacle, and by learning to use weakness instead of allowing weakness to govern her behavior.

7. The ability to develop interpersonal relationships.

8. Positive self-image characteristics of the successful medical assistant include:
    A. Identifying with people.
    B. Feeling personally and mentally adequate.
    C. Having the ability to organize her life.
    D. Being dependable and reliable.
    E. Being professionally needed and valued.
    F. Being concerned with the needs of others.
    G. Being attractive and likeable.

Pretest
Answer Key

---

9. The medical assistant should be more concerned with patient care than with office procedures, rules, or regulations. The patient's needs and experiences should have priority over objective facts, charts, or office rules and regulations.

10. A proper appearance creates a good first impression and gives the medical assistant an opportunity to demonstrate her strengths and assets. Physical health and physical energy are closely related; hence, a medical assistant should practice good personal hygiene along with some type of physical exercise program and eat a well-balanced diet.

11. The successful medical assistant possesses the mental capacity to learn the necessary technical skills. She is organized, yet flexible, and not afraid of changes in office procedures. She possess personal initiative and foresight. She is able to display a degree of toughness and tenderness at the same time; she understands the impact of what she does and says and is personally responsible for her actions. The successful medical assistant is patient.

12. A pleasant smile builds another person's confidence in the smiling person because the smile suggests that the person has her life under control. At the same time, it builds confidence in the person to whom the smile is directed because it encourages his personal worth. Smiling has a mushrooming effect because it passes so easily for person to person. A smile is the most influential social skill a person can possess.

13. A good conversationalist encourages other people to talk about themselves. She talks about herself only at another's invitation. The good conversationalist talks of cheerful matters, not personal burdens. She does not tease and is not sarcastic; rather, she has developed the art of being a good listener.

14. The patient's name.

15. First Stage: Denial—The patient doesn't admit the reality of the diagnosis.
    Second Stage: Anger—The patient is bitter and hostile.
    Third Stage: Bargaining—The patient practices good behavior seeking the reward of an extension on life.
    Fourth Stage: Depression—The patient faces reality of the many losses he will endure and prepares himself for these losses.
    Fifth Stage: Acceptance—The patient becomes calm and develops a readiness to die.

16. When a person is struggling with a particular problem, the struggle will affect how she handles other matters and deals with other people and vice versa. Therefore, if the medical assistant has a problem in the office, she should involve co-workers and the physician-employer in analyzing and solving the problem since it will affect them as well.

17. Begin with a positive statement. Then focus on the inappropriateness of the behavior, rather than the person. Know what the person did wrong and be prepared to tell him how to do it right. Remember, criticism does not have to be repeated. End the discussion in a positive fashion.

Personal Practice Learning Activities

Many people who seek personal counseling are searching for answers to the following questions: Who am I? Where am I going? Do I have any control over how I get there? Everyone is searching for an identity. We all have an identity, however, some people are unaware of or deny their identity. The following activities are designed to assist you in becoming acquainted with yourself and more aware of your relationships with others.

1. Name Tag

    A. Write the name you most like to be called in the middle of your name tag.

<table>
<tr><td>1. ____________</td><td>1. ____________</td></tr>
<tr><td>2. ____________</td><td>2. ____________</td></tr>
<tr><td>3. ____________</td><td>3. ____________</td></tr>
<tr><td>4. ____________</td><td>4. ____________</td></tr>
<tr><td colspan="2" align="center">________</td></tr>
<tr><td>1. ____________</td><td>1. ____________</td></tr>
<tr><td>2. ____________</td><td>2. ____________</td></tr>
<tr><td>3. ____________</td><td>3. ____________</td></tr>
<tr><td>4. ____________</td><td>4. ____________</td></tr>
</table>

    B. In the upper left-hand corner write the names of four unrelated people who have had the most influences on your life.

    C. In the lower left-hand corner list four geographical locations (cities, states, lakes, etc.) that are especially meaningful to you.

    D. On line 1, in the upper right-hand corner, write the name of the person you would call first if you needed help. On line 2, write the feeling you would have if you were paged while attending a football game. On line 3, write the date of the last time you cried. On line 4, write the date of the last time you said "I love you" to someone.

**Personal Practice
Learning Activities**

E. In the lower right-hand corner on line 1, describe an activity that you learned very easily. On line 2 describe an activity that you found very difficult to learn. On line 3, describe something you would like to change, and on line 4, cite one idea you have gained from this activity.

F. Examine your name tag.

   1) What have you learned about yourself?

   2) What feeling do you have right now?

   3) How would you feel about sharing your name tag with others?

G. The next time you are responsible for helping a group become acquainted, you might try a similar activity. After everyone has completed his or her name tag, form small groups to discuss the topics in each corner. Form new groups each time you move from corner to corner of the name tag.

2. Open-ended statements.

   A. Complete each sentence.

      1) I am happy when

      2) I like people who

      3) My best friend is

      4) My job is

      5) Patients are

      6) The best thing that could happen to me is

      7) I am proud when I

      8) I feel best when I

      9) When I'm not working, I like to

      10) I wish somebody knew that I

Personal Practice
Learning Activities

B. After completing the ten previous sentences, answer the following:

1) I learned that I

2) I wish that I had

3) I hope I will

4) I am

5) I will

3. Feeling words

A. List as many words as you can that describe the various feelings you had during the last day you worked.

B. Answer the following questions:

1) In general, were your feelings more positive or more negative?

2) Who influenced you to feel as you did?

3) What are the characteristics of a positive relationship?

4) How did you influence others to feel as they did?

5) What did you do that caused others to respond to you as they did?

6) What did you like best about your day?

7) What did you like least about your day?

8) What could you have done to improve your day?

**Personal Practice
Learning Activities**

---

4. What I do for fun

    A. List things you like to do, big or little, personal or job related, as long as they are important to you.

Important Activities	1	2	3	4	5	6	7	8
1.								
2.								
3.								
4.								
5.								
6.								
7.								
8.								
9.								
10.								
11.								
12.								
13.								
14.								
15.								
16.								
17.								
18.								
19.								
20.								

Personal Practice
Learning Activities

B. In column 1, place an A after each activity you prefer doing alone or an O after those activities you prefer doing with others. Place an AO if it doesn't matter. Add an F if this activity includes your family.

C. In column 2, place a $ after each activity costing more than $5 to do.

D. In column 3, place a check (√) after those activities you do daily, an X after those activities you do weekly, and the date you last did the others.

E. In column 4, place a C after those activities you have done since childhood, a P after those activities you have been doing for less than two years, and an R after those activities you hope to still be doing during retirement.

F. In column 5, place a PH after those activities that involve physical exercise, an I after those that are intellectual, and an ART after those that are artistic.

G. In column 6, place a PR after those activities in which you are an active participant and a PS after those that require you to be a spectator.

H. In column 7, place an RX after those activities that are for relaxation and an SI after those that are for self-improvement.

I. In column 8, place an MO after those activities you would like to do more often.

J. Look at your chart. Consider the following questions:

1) What does this data suggest? What have you learned about yourself?

2) Do you see any patterns or trends?

3) Are you more of a loner or a person who does things with others?

**Personal Practice
Learning Activities**

---

    4)   Are you a doer or an observer?

    5)   Does your fun cost a lot of money?

    6)   Are you taking time for fun?

K. After answering the six previous questions, complete the following sentences.

    1)   I was surprised that I

    2)   I was saddened that I

    3)   I enjoyed

    4)   I plan to change

5. Strengths and weaknesses

Each of us has strengths and weaknesses, assets and liabilities, and talents and skills that influence who and what we are. That we have certain strengths and/or weaknesses is not as important as how we choose to use them. This activity is designed to help you get in touch with your personal and professional strengths and weaknesses.

**Personal Practice
Learning Activities**

A. List your strengths and weaknesses.

        Strengths   Weaknesses

B. Answer the following questions:

1) How are you taking advantage of your strengths?

2) How do you let your weaknesses control what you do or do not do?

3) Are you so concerned with overcoming your weaknesses that you forget to utilize your strong points? Explain how you do this or keep from doing it.

4) How might your life or your job change if you concerned yourself only with your strengths?

Post-Test   As concisely as possible, answer each of the following questions without referring to your book or other material. When finished, refer to the Chapter III post-test answer key.

1. A person's self-concept consists of:

2. Explain the relationship between feedback and self-concept.

3. How can feedback cause a conflict between the real and ideal self?

4. List four ways to promote your self-concept.

5. Discuss how a person can minimize her weaknesses.

6. Who and what determine the degree of happiness, success, joy, and fulfillment an individual receives from life?

7. In addition to adequate knowledge and technical skill, what is an essential ingredient for being a successful medical assistant?

Post-Test

---

8. How does the successful medical assistant usually feel about physicians, co-workers, and patients?

9. Explain the importance of a well-balanced personal life to one's work as a medical assistant.

10. Describe the mental characteristics of a successful medical assistant.

11. Explain the effect a smile has on other people.

12. What are the characteristics of a good conversationalist?

13. Identify and explain the four elements in the 4-A Formula for developing social skills.

14. List and briefly describe the five stages of dying as classified by Elisabeth Kübler-Ross, MD.

15. Briefly discuss how to use the effective method when criticism is necessary.

**Post-Test
Answer Key**

Compare your answers to the post-test questions to the correct answers given in the following key. While your response to each question need not correspond exactly with the words used in the answers below, the meanings must be similar in order for your response to be considered correct.

If you answer eleven of the fifteen questions correctly, you will have demonstrated a satisfactory understanding of the material in Chapter III and should proceed to the Personal Practice Learning Activities if you have not completed them or to Chapter IV if you have. If you answer fewer than eleven questions correctly, you should restudy the appropriate sections of Chapter III before proceeding with the Activities or Chapter IV.

---

1. A person's self-concept consists of all the beliefs and attitudes he has about himself—in other words, how he sees himself.

2. Feedback is the reaction a person receives from another as a result of a certain behavior. Positive reactions to behavior improve a person's self-concept while negative reactions hurt or damage one's self-concept.

3. If the feedback received is not compatible with what is desired or believed, a conflict develops between the real and ideal self. How one responds to feedback determines whether one remains as is, regresses, or grows as a person.

4. You can promote your self-concept by:

   A. Being open and honest with yourself and others.
   B. Speaking and operating from the positive.
   C. Practicing positive communication skills.
   D. Developing an "I'm OK" attitude.

5. By concentrating on her strengths and those things she does well, a person can minimize her weaknesses. She should accept weakness as a challenge rather than considering it an obstacle, and she should learn to use weaknesses rather than allowing weaknesses to govern her behavior.

6. The individual and the way she feels about herself and others.

7. The ability to develop interpersonal relationships.

8. The successful medical assistant feels that physicians, co-workers, and patients deserve respect, and she sees them as individuals capable of finding solutions for their own problems while possessing dignity, infinite worth and value.

Post-Test
Answer Key

---

9. A medical assistant's personal life is disclosed through her attitudes toward her job. Personal problems that are allowed to go unsolved reduce her ability to concentrate on her work with physicians, co-workers, and patients.

10. The successful medical assistant possesses the mental capacity to learn the necessary technical skills. She is organized, yet flexible, and not afraid of changes in office procedures. She possesses personal initiative and foresight. She is able to display a degree of toughness and tenderness at the same time; she understands the impact of what she does and says and is personally responsible for her actions. The successful medical assistant is patient.

11. A pleasant smile builds another person's confidence in the smiling person because the smile suggests that the person has her life under control. At the same time, it builds confidence in the person whom the smile is directed because it encourages his personal worth. Smiling has a mushrooming effect because it passes so easily from person to person. A smile is the most influential social skill a person can possess.

12. A good conversationalist encourages other people to talk about themselves. She talks about herself only at another's invitation. The good conversationalist talks of cheerful matters, not personal burdens. She does not tease and is not sarcastic; rather, she has developed the art of being a good listener.

13. The 4-A formula:
    A. *Accept* people as they are.
    B. Find something to *approve* in the other person.
    C. Show sincere *appreciation,* thereby raising the other person's opinion of herself.
    D. Exhibit an attitude of *affirmation,* thereby creating a positive atmosphere for the people around you.

14. First Stage: Denial—The patient does not admit the reality of the diagnosis.
    Second Stage: Anger—The patient is bitter and hostile.
    Third Stage: Bargaining—The patient practices good behavior seeking the reward of an extension on life.
    Fourth Stage: Depression—The patient faces the reality of the many losses he will endure and prepares himself for those losses.
    Fifth Stage: Acceptance—The patient becomes calm and develops a readiness to die.

15. Begin with a positive statement. Then focus on the inappropriateness of the behavior, rather than the person. Know what the person did wrong and be prepared to tell him how to do it right. Remember, criticism does not have to be repeated, so only one criticism per behavior is sufficient. End the discussion in a positive fashion.

Related Readings

1. Allen J. *As a Man Thinketh.* Lakemont, Ga: CSA Press; 1975.

2. Carnegie D. *How to Win Friends and Influence People.* New York, NY: Simon & Schuster; 1936.

3. Clason G. *The Richest Man in Babylon.* New York, NY: Hawthorn Books Inc; 1955.

4. Gibran K. *The Prophet.* New York, NY: Alfred A Knopf Inc; 1923.

5. Glasser W. *Positive Addiction.* New York, NY: Harper & Row Publishers; 1976.

6. Jourard S. *The Transparent Self.* 2nd ed. New York, NY: Van Nostrand Reinhold; 1971.

7. Selye H. *The Stress of Life.* New York, NY: McGraw-Hill Book Company Inc; 1956.

8. Shostrom E. *Man, The Manipulator.* Nashville, Tenn: Abingdon Press; 1967.

9. Simon S. *Meeting Yourself Halfway.* Chicago, Ill: Argus Communications; 1974.

10. Yamamoto K (ed). *The Child and His Image. Boston,* Mass: Houghton Mifflin Co; 1972.

Additional readings

Boffey B. *Reinventing Yourself.* Chapel Hill, NC: New View Publications; 1993.

Chopra D. *The Seven Spiritual Laws of Success.* San Rafael, Calif: Amber-Allen; 1994.

Good E. *In Pursuit of Happiness.* Chapel Hill, NC: New View Publications; 1987.

Goulston M and Goldberg P. *Get Out Of Your Own Way.* New York, NY: Penguin Putnam; 1996.

Johnson S. *Who Moved My Cheese.* New York, NY: G.P. Putnam's Sons; 1998.

Moore T. *Care of the Soul.* New York, NY: Harper Collins Publishers, Inc; 1992.

Chapter IV:

How do we communicate?

   Remember to allow time to discuss related reading done by a group
member and any troublesome Post-Test questions.

1. From the book:

    A. Review the chapter objectives and competency checks.
    B. Discuss the nature of interpersonal communications.
    C. Discuss the unproductive communication styles.
    D. Discuss the barriers to positive relationships.

2. From the workbook:

    A. Activities 1 and 3 can be done during class, with the results discussed.
    B. Activities 2, 4, and 5 should be done prior to class, with small groups formed to discuss the
       results during class.
    C. If time is limited, Activities 2 and 4 should be given priority during class.

Pretest   In the space provided answer concisely each of the following questions. The answer key follows the pretest.

1. Define communications.

2. What is the principal difference between conversing and communicating?

3. List the four major factors affecting the communication process.

4. Most of a person's communication is determined by which important characteristic?

5. An individual with an extremely low, negative self-image could be classified as what kind of person?

6. Differentiate between the fence rider and the pretender.

7. Explain why a person might become too involved in the minute details of a particular event.

Pretest

---

8. In a medical office why is the so-called "expert" a potentially dangerous person?

9. Analyze the effect a command such as "Stop complaining and give me the patient's record" could have on the co-worker receiving the message.

10. State the principal difference between lecturing and threatening.

11. How can interpreting be a barrier to positive communication?

12. Contrast the barrier of sympathizing to the barrier of humoring.

Pretest
Answer Key

Compare your responses to the pretest questions to the correct answers stated in the following key. If you answer nine of the twelve questions correctly, proceed to the Personal Practice Learning Activities, as you have successfully challenged the content of this chapter. If fewer than nine of your answers are correct, you should study the material in Chapter IV of the book.

Your answers need not correspond exactly to the answers in the key below, but the meanings of the two responses must be similar in order for your answer to be considered correct.

---

1. Communication is a process of interaction by which human beings relate to each other. The process requires the use of symbols—verbal and nonverbal—which act as stimuli to evoke a reply in another person.

2. When communicating, people are engaged in the process of trying to understand each other; when conversing, the participants usually are engaged in the process of self-enhancement or self-maintenance.

3. The four major factors affecting the communication process:

   A. The shared goals of task completing and group maintenance.
   B. The emotions and feelings of people involved in the process.
   C. Diverse group and individual purposes, both obvious and concealed.
   D. The diversity of verbal and nonverbal symbols.

4. The desire to protect, maintain, and enhance her self-image.

5. A defensive person.

6. The fence rider is a very cool, calm and collected individual who is quite sophisticated and seldom shows any emotions. She never volunteers information and tends to talk out of both sides of her mouth when a conflicts arises. The pretender differs to the extreme in that she may be considered a phony. She is rebellious, resistive and so uninterested in what is going on that she never deals with conflicts or issues in the office. She ignores all situations and is usually out of touch with other people.

7. A person may become too involved in the facts and figures of a situation in order to avoid dealing with feelings and emotions or to hide her own emotions and feelings.

8. The so-called "expert" can be very dangerous because she has a tendency to offer patients medical advice which is not legitimate or valid.

9. This command could produce fear and resistance and would likely prompt retaliative and rebellious behavior in the co-worker.

Pretest
Answer Key

10. Lecturing refers to telling another person through persuasion, logic, or argument how a situation is going to be; threatening refers to warning or promising another person what the consequences of an action or inaction will be.

11. Listening to another person "diagnose" or "interpret" one's motives or actions can be threatening and frustrating and may stop communication with the interpreter for fear of being exposed as a weak person.

12. Sympathizing refers to trying to make another person feel better by using a serious method to talk her out of her feelings or to make feelings go away. In contrast, humoring is an attempt to divert the person's attention from the problem in a jocular or less serious way.

Personal Practice
Learning Activities

---

1. Recognizing unproductive communication styles

    Match each of the statements listed on the right with one of the unproductive communication styles listed on the left.

    A. Offensive   _____ 1. "Well, I just don't know."

    B. Defensive   _____ 2. "Blue Cross wants it done like this"

    C. Fence Rider   _____ 3. "This is really a bum typewriter."

    D. Pretender   _____ 4. "I want you to do it this way."

    E. Sweet Talker   _____ 5. "What did you say to that?"

    F. Prober   _____ 6. "Why, you must be the best doctor in town!"

    G. Expert   _____ 7. "You're so right; whatever you say, I'll do."

    H. Critic   _____ 8. "Anyone for bingo tonight?"

The correct answers are on page 74.

2. Responding to communication styles

    A. List three incidences in which a physician related to you using one of the unproductive communication styles.

        1) How did you feel? Describe your emotions at the time.

        2) How did you respond to the physician? What did you do as a result of how he related to you?

**Personal Practice
Learning Activities**

---

    3) What did you learn about *yourself* in regard to communication styles?

B. List three incidences in which a colleague related to you using one of the unproductive communication styles.

    1) How did you feel? Describe your emotions at the time.

    2) How did you respond to the colleague? What did you do as a result of how she related to you?

    3) What did you learn about *yourself* in regard to communication styles?

C. List three incidences from your personal life where a friend or relative related to you using one of the unproductive communication styles.

    1) How did you feel? Describe your emotions at the time.

**Personal Practice
Learning Activities**

---

    2) How did you respond to your friend? What did you do as a result of how he/she related to you?

    3) What did you learn about *yourself* in regard to communication styles?

D. List three incidences from your personal or professional life where you used one of the unproductive communication styles to related to another person.

    1) How did you feel? Describe your emotions at the time.

    2) How did the other person respond? How did you respond to the other person's response?

    3) What did you learn about yourself in regard to unproductive communication styles?

Personal Practice
Learning Activities

---

3. Recognizing barriers to positive relationships

    Match each of the statements on the right with one of the barriers on the left.

    A. Advising   _______   1.   "You should wear warmer clothing."

    B. Commanding   _______   2.   "You're probably catching a cold."

    C. Criticizing   _______   3.   "You're always complaining about something."

    D. Humoring   _______   4.   "If you don't quit worrying about the little things, you're going to lose some patients."

    E. Interpreting   _______   5.   "Oh, you poor thing! I'll bet you're coming down with something."

    F. Interrogating   _______   6.   "You should be pleased. We are saving on the heating bill. Energy, too!"

    G. Lecturing   _______   7.   "Don't worry about the cold. Think of the patients."

    H. Shaming   _______   8.   "Well, at least you're healthy."

    I. Sympathizing   _______   9.   "What temperature do you keep your thermostat on at home?"

    J. Threatening   _______   10.   "You know the saying, 'Cold nose, healthy body.'"

The correct answers are on page 74.

4. Barrier awareness and effects

    A. List all the barriers that you remember being used by the physicians in the three incidences recorded in Activity 2A.

    1) How did you feel? Describe your emotional reactions to the barriers.

    2) How did you respond to the barriers?

**Personal Practice
Learning Activities**

---

    3) What have you learned about barriers to positive relationships?

B. List all the barriers that you remember being used by the colleagues in the three incidences recorded in Activity 2B.

    1) How did you feel? Describe your emotional reactions to the barriers.

    2) How did you respond to the barriers?

    3) What have you learned about barriers to positive relationships?

C. List all the barriers that you remember being used by your friends or relatives in the three incidences recorded in Activity 2C.

    1) How did you feel? Describe your emotional reactions to the barriers.

---

2) How did you respond to the barriers?

3) What have you learned about barriers to positive relationships?

D. List all the barriers that you remember using in the three incidences recorded in Activity 2D.

1) How did you feel?

2) What response did you receive most often? How did you feel about the response?

3) What have you learned about barriers to positive relationships?

Personal Practice
Learning Activities

---

5. Observing and recording interactions

    On a daily basis for one working week, observe and record all examples of unproductive communication styles and barriers to positive relationships between the following persons.

    A. Monday:

        1) Physician to you

        2) Colleague to you

        3) Physician to patient

        4) Colleague to patient

        5) You to physician

        6) You to colleague

**Personal Practice
Learning Activities**

---

    7) You to patient

    8) Record all the emotions you felt during the day.

    9) How did your feelings about the interactions affect your work day?

    10) What did you learn about communications today?

B. Tuesday:

    1) Physician to you

    2) Colleague to you

    3) Physician to patient

**Personal Practice
Learning Activities**

---

4) Colleague to patient

5) You to physician

6) You to colleague

7) You to patient

8) Record all the emotions you felt during the day.

9) How did your feelings about the interactions affect your work day?

10) What did you learn about communications today?

**Personal Practice
Learning Activities**

C. Wednesday:

1) Physician to you

2) Colleague to you

3) Physician to patient

4) Colleague to patient

5) You to physician

6) You to colleague

7) You to patient

**Personal Practice
Learning Activities**

---

8) Record all the emotions you felt during the day.

9) How did your feelings about the interactions affect your work day?

10) What did you learn about communications today?

D. Thursday:

1) Physician to you

2) Colleague to you

3) Physician to patient

4) Colleague to patient

**Personal Practice
Learning Activities**

---

5) You to physician

6) You to colleague

7) You to patient

8) Record all the emotions you felt during the day.

9) How did your feelings about the interactions affect your work day?

10) What did you learn about communications today?

E. Friday:

1) Physician to you

**Personal Practice
Learning Activities**

---

2) Colleague to you

3) Physician to patient

4) Colleague to patient

5) You to physician

6) You to colleague

7) You to patient

8) Record all the emotions you felt during the day.

**Personal Practice
Learning Activities**

---

9) How did your feelings about the interactions affect your work day?

10) What did you learn about communications today?

F. Summary

Complete the following statements:

1) I learned that I

2) I am pleased that I

3) I regret that I

4) I hope that I

**Personal Practice
Learning Activities**

Check your answers to Activities 1 and 3 with the key below.

---

1. Activity 1: Recognizing unproductive communication styles

    C-1   A-4   B-7
    G-2   F-5   D-8
    H-2   E-6

2. Activity 3: Recognizing barriers to positive relationships

    A-1   I-5   F-9
    E-2   G-6   D-10
    C-3   B-7
    J-4   H-8

Post-Test As concisely as possible, answer each of the following questions without referring to your book or other material. When finished, refer to the Chapter IV post-test answer key.

---

1. Why is the ability to communicate effectively essential for the medical assistant?

2. Describe two variables that influence any communication interaction.

3. Most of a person's communication is determined by which important characteristic?

4. Describe the offensive person.

5. From a communication standpoint discuss the behavior of a sweet talker.

6. Explain how a critic might be detrimental to the office environment.

7. In the communication process, what effect does advising have on the receiver?

Post-Test

---

8. Which of the barriers would best describe the following statement: "You're not thinking clearly today; the patient's record should have been completely this way."

9. How can sympathizing be a barrier to positive relationships?

10. How does the prober differ from the interrogator?

11. List the ten barriers to positive relationships.

12. List eight common unproductive communication styles.

**Post-Test
Answer Key**

Compare your answers to the post-test questions to the correct answers given in the following key. While your response to each question need not correspond exactly with the words used in the answers below, the meanings must be similar in order for your response to be considered correct.

If you answer nine of the twelve questions correctly, you will have demonstrated a satisfactory understanding of the material in Chapter IV and should proceed to the Personal Practice Learning Activities if you have not completed them or to Chapter V if you have. If you answer fewer than nine questions correctly, you should restudy the appropriate sections of Chapter IV before proceeding.

1. Effective communication is essential for the welfare of patients.

2. The physical and emotional selves of participants in the communication interaction.

3. The desire to protect, maintain, and enhance her self-image.

4. The offensive person usually has a tough, dictatorial, authoritative, dominating and superior manner. She is disagreeable, skeptical, eager to assign blame, a poor listener, and insensitive to other people. Beneath this facade is a very insecure and scared individual.

5. The sweet talker uses gushy, flowery phrases and is reluctant to conform or share her feelings about any unpleasant topic. She tends to compliment everyone and everything. She sweet talks and butters up people in order to maintain her position and security.

6. Criticism of the office, including procedures, policies, staff, and service, may be overheard by patients, resulting in a loss of confidence and trust and creating doubt about the quality of care provided.

7. Advising tends to make the receiver feel insecure about her ability to solve a problem or make a decision.

8. The barrier of criticizing.

9. Sympathizing can be a barrier to positive relationships because it tends to ignore or deny the other person's feeling, and this often causes the recipient of the sympathy to feel that she was not understood.

10. The prober asks questions to avoid dealing with emotion surrounding a case; the interrogator asks questions to solve another person's problem rather than assisting the other person to solve the problem herself.

Post-Test
Answer Key

---

11. The ten barriers to positive relationships are:

1) commanding	4) lecturing	7) interpreting
2) threatening	5) criticizing	8) sympathizing
3) advising	6) shaming	9) interrogating
		10) humoring

12. Eight unproductive communication styles:

1) offensive person	5) sweet talker
2) defensive person	6) prober
3) fence rider	7) expert
4) pretender	8) critic

Related readings

---

1. Carkhuff R. *The Art of Helping.* Amherst, Mass: Human Resource Development Press Inc; 1973.

2. Gaulke E. *You Can Have a Family Where Everybody Wins.* St. Louis, Mo: Concordia Publishing House; 1975.

3. Ginott H. *Between Parent & Child.* New York, NY: MacMillan Co; 1965.

4. Gordon A. *A Touch of Wonder.* Carmel, NY: Fleming H Revell Cl Inc; 1974.

5. Johnson D, Johnson R. *Learning Together and Alone.* Englewood Cliffs, NJ: Prentice-Hall Inc; 1975.

6. Johnson D. *Reaching Out.* Englewood Cliffs, NJ: Prentice-Hall Inc; 1972.

7. Miller S, Nunnally E, Wakeman D. *Alive and Aware.* Minneapolis, Minn: Interpersonal Communications Program Inc; 1975.

8. Powel J. *Why Am I Afraid to Tell You Who I Am?* Chicago, Ill: Argus Communications; 1969.

Additional readings

Brown H. *Life's Little Instruction Book.* Nashville, Tenn: Rutlege Hill Press; 1991.

Jackson P, Delehunty H. *Sacred Hoops.* New York, NY: Hyperion; 1995.

Kushner H. *When Bad Things Happen to Good People.* New York, NY: Schocken Books; 1981.

Richardson C. *Take Time For Your Life.* New York, NY: Broadway Books; 1999.

Richardson C. *Life Makeovers.* New York, NY: Broadway Brooks; 2000.

Chapter V:

Healthy relationships

**Guidelines for
Group Study**

---

1. From the book:

    A. Review the chapter objectives and competency check questions.
    B. Discuss the notion of healthy relationships.
    C. Discuss the essential ingredients of healthy relationships.
    D. Discuss and give examples of the basic skills that facilitate the Effective Communication System.
    E. Discuss each of the ten steps of the problem-solving model.

2. From the workbook:

    A. Activities 1 and 2 are not recommended for group meetings.
    B. Activity 3 should be completed prior to class, with small groups formed to discuss the responses during class.
    C. Activity 4 should be completed prior to class. During class each group member should choose one situation with a physician, one with a colleague, and one with a patient or friend and share the situation and her responses with other group members.
    D. Activity 5 can be done in a number of ways:
        1) The activity can be completed prior to class, with each group member sharing one of the situations and her problem-solving approach with other members in the small group. The group members should be able to clarify and offer helpful suggestions to the individual.
        2) The group may want to solve a common problem utilizing the ten-step approach to problem solving.
        3) Specific problem situations may be selected, with group members role-playing the characters involved.

Pretest   In the space provided answer concisely each of the following questions. The answer key follows the pretest.

---

1. How can a medical assistant improve her interpersonal relationships?

2. Contrasts the accepting to the unaccepting medical assistant.

3. An empathetic person has the ability to:

4. Why is the concrete medical assistant an asset to the medical office?

5. Define immediacy as used in the Effective Communication System.

6. Briefly describe the potent medical assistant.

7. State the principal difference between silence and listening.

Pretest

---

8. Why is perception-checking an important listening sub-skill?

9. When during the communication process should feedback be given?

10. Define assertiveness.

11. List the ten steps to problem solving.

12. Why is the ten-step problem-solving model valuable to the medical assistant?

**Pretest
Answer Key**

Compare your responses to the pretest questions to the correct answers stated in the following key. If you answer nine of the twelve questions correctly, proceed to the Personal Practice Learning Activities, as you have successfully challenged the content of this chapter. If fewer than nine of your answers are correct, you should study the material in Chapter V of the book.

Your answers need not correspond exactly to the answers in the key, but the meanings of the two responses must be similar in order for your answer to be considered correct.

---

1. A medical assistant can improve interpersonal relationships by developing a positive language of acceptance.

2. The accepting medical assistant addresses herself to an individual's situation. The unaccepting medical assistant judges the individual's character and personality.

3. An empathetic person can perceive and understand another individual's situation and communicate that understanding to the individual.

4. The concrete medical assistant is an asset to the medical office because she helps people identify and talk about their feelings instead of speculating or gossiping about other people and events. She relates to people in a way that encourages concreteness from them.

5. Immediacy is the ability to deal with what is going on right now. Immediacy is dealing with your feeling toward the patient, physician, or colleague with regard to what is happening at the moment.

6. The potent medical assistant is interested in, concerned about, and involved in the health-care delivery of the total office.

7. Silence is basically nonverbal listening when no verbal response is required. Listening is understanding *and* responding to the total message being sent; the response may be verbal or nonverbal but will somehow let the other person know that the message has been received and understood.

8. Perception-checking gives the listener an opportunity to verify her perception of what is being said, thereby avoiding misunderstandings and hurt feelings.

9. Feedback should be given as soon as possible after the behavior that evokes the feedback and when both individuals are emotionally prepared and have the time to discuss and process the information.

10. Assertiveness is expressing yourself in such a manner that your needs, wants, thoughts, feelings and desires are known to another person.

Pretest
Answer Key

---

11. The ten steps to problem solving:

   1) Identify the problem.
   2) Analyze your role in the problem.
   3) Diagnose the results of your past behavior.
   4) Clarify your goals.
   5) Prescribe the treatment plan.
   6) Implement treatment strategy.
   7) Observe the treatment-strategy consequences.
   8) Evaluate the treatment-strategy results.
   9) Maintain or modify the treatment plan.
   10) Review and/or repeat the process.

12. The ten-step problem-solving model provides the medical assistant with a systematic way of arranging her thoughts and resources so that she can successfully solve problems and cope with conflicts.

**Personal Practice
Learning Activities**

---

1. Essential ingredients

    Observe and record interactions at home and work that demonstrate each of the eight essential ingredients in the Effective Communication System. Remember, interactions may be verbal or nonverbal. Record who did or said what to whom for each ingredient.

    A. Empathy

      1. Home:

      2. Work:

    B. Respect

      1. Home:

      2. Work:

    C. Genuineness

      1. Home:

      2. Work:

Personal Practice
Learning Activities

    D. Concreteness

        1. Home:

        2. Work:

    E.   Self-Disclosure

        1. Home:

        2. Work:

    F.   Confrontation

        1. Home:

        2. Work:

**Personal Practice
Learning Activities**

   G. Immediacy

      1. Home:

      2. Work:

   H. Potency

      1. Home:

      2. Work:

Personal Practice
Learning Activities

---

2. Recognizing effective responses

   Match the following communication skills with the appropriate statement listed below. The correct answers are on page 104.

   A. Open-ended acknowledgment
   B. Effective listening
   C. Paraphrasing

   D. Perception-checking
   E. Feedback
   F. Assertiveness

   ___ 1) "You want me to file the report from Dr. Jones after I make copies for Drs. Smith, Kelly and Johnson?"

   ___ 2) "I really get nervous when you stand over my shoulder watching me type, and it causes me to make more errors."

   ___ 3) "You feel hurried and pressured when I schedule patients so close together, and you would like me to give you more time."

   ___ 4) "I would like to hear how you would handle this situation."

   ___ 5) "When you call to tell me that you have an emergency at the hospital and will be 20 minutes late, it really helps me to be able to inform patients to that effect. They feel less irritated."

   ___ 6) "You are pretty irritated with Mrs. Porter for not following her diet."

3. Effective listening

   Write an effective listening response to the statements listed on the succeeding pages. Remember to respond to the feelings the person is having. We suggest beginning each of your responses with "You feel..." to help you focus on the emotions as well as the content or facts of the situation. Once, however, you develop the art of responding to both feelings and facts, you will alter the sentence structure of your responses. Beginning every sentence with "You feel" would become redundant. Remember, too, that this is your first response to an expressed concern and will probably be only one of several that you will make regarding a particular situation.

   When finished with this activity, compare the feeling words used in your response with those suggested on page 104.

   Example: Patient says, "I have been waiting over an hour to see Dr. Smith. How much longer will it be?"

   You respond, "You feel pretty irritated with having to wait so long and wish you could get in and get it over with."

**Personal Practice
Learning Activities**

A. Physician says, "I do not want to go to that meeting on Saturday. Johnny and I had planned to go fishing."

    You respond, "You feel …

B. Patient says, "When you get old, you expect all sorts of accidents. Guess I am lucky it was not worse."

    You respond, "You feel …

C. Colleague says, "I just do not understand what Dr. Jones wants from me. I am doing the best I can."

    You respond, "You feel …

D. Physician says, "I wanted to go to medical school and be a doctor more than anything in the world, but some days I wonder if I made the right choice."

    You respond, "You feel …

E. Patient says, "Can you get the doctor to give me something stronger for this pain?"
    You respond, "You feel …

**Personal Practice
Learning Activities**

F.   Colleague says, "Jim and I decided last night to get a divorce."
     You respond, "You feel …

G.   Physician says, "Aren't those lab reports back yet? What do those people do all day?"
     You respond, "You feel …

H.   Patient says, "I just don't know what I'll do. Everything is so expensive, and we do not have any insurance."
     You respond, "You feel …

I.   Colleague says, "I feel more like an errand girl around here than a medical assistant."
     You respond, "You feel …

J.   Patient says, "You are different from most medical people. You seem to care about me as a person."
     You respond, "You feel …

**Personal Practice
Learning Activities**

---

4. Effective assertiveness

Think of situations where physicians, colleagues, patients, and friends behave in ways that either please you or cause you concern. For each situation describe the behavior, your feelings, and the behavior's effect on you in the spaces below, and then write an appropriately assertive response summing up the situation. An example of an appropriately assertive response:

> "When you keep me after quitting time to take dictation, I get nervous and upset and cannot do my best work. Also, I ride in a car pool, and the other riders should not have to wait for me."

After writing your assertive response, make plans to actually use the message.

A. Situation 1

    1) Physician's behavior:

    2) Your feeling:

    3) Effect on you:

    4) Your response:

B. Situation 2

    1) Physician's behavior:

    2) Your feeling:

Personal Practice
Learning Activities

---

    3) Effect on you:

    4) Your response:

C. Situation 3

    1) Physician's behavior:

    2) Your feeling:

    3) Effect on you:

    4) Your response:

D. Situation 4

    1) Colleague's behavior:

    2) Your feeling:

    3) Effect on you:

**Personal Practice
Learning Activities**

---

    4) Your response:

  E. Situation 5

    1) Colleague's behavior:

    2) Your feeling:

    3) Effect on you:

    4) Your response:

  F. Situation 6

    1) Colleague's behavior:

    2) Your feeling:

    3) Effect on you:

    4) Your response:

Personal Practice
Learning Activities

G. Situation 7

   1) Patient's behavior:

   2) Your feeling:

   3) Effect on you:

   4) Your response:

H. Situation 8

   1) Patient's behavior:

   2) Your feeling:

   3) Effect on you:

   4) Your response:

**Personal Practice
Learning Activities**

I. Situation 9

   1) Patient's behavior:

   2) Your feeling:

   3) Effect on you:

   4) Your response:

J. Situation 10

   1) Friend's behavior:

   2) Your feeling:

   3) Effect on you:

   4) Your response:

Personal Practice
Learning Activities

K. Situation 11
   1) Friend's behavior:

   2) Your feeling:

   3) Effect on you:

   4) Your response:

L. Situation 12
   1) Friend's behavior:

   2) Your feeling:

   3) Effect on you:

   4) Your response:

**Personal Practice
Learning Activities**

---

5. Problem solving

   Identify four situations in your personal and professional life which cause you some dissatisfaction. Consider your unmet needs and conflicts with others. Describe the problem and then complete the details for the ten steps of the problem-solving model.

   A. Situation 1 (Describe a problem with a physician)

   Step 1. *Identify* the problem:

   Step 2. *Analyze* your role:

   Step 3. *Diagnose* the result of past behavior:

   Step 4. *Clarify* your goals:

   Step 5. *Prescribe* treatment:

   Step 6. *Implement* treatment strategy:

Personal Practice
Learning Activities

Step 7. *Observe* consequences of treatment:

Step 8. *Evaluate* results:

Step 9. *Maintain* or *Modify* plan:

Step 10. *Review* and/or *Repeat:*

B. Situation 2 (Describe a problem with a colleague)

Step 1. *Identify* the problem:

Step 2. *Analyze* your role:

Step 3. *Diagnose* the results of past behavior:

**Personal Practice
Learning Activities**

Step 4. *Clarify* your goals:

Step 5. *Prescribe* treatment:

Step 6. *Implement* treatment strategy:

Step 7. *Observe* consequences of treatment:

Step 8. *Evaluate* results:

Step 9. *Maintain* or *Modify* plan:

Step 10. *Review* and/or *Repeat:*

**Personal Practice
Learning Activities**

C. Situation 3 (Describe a problem with a patient)

Step 1. *Identify* the problem:

Step 2. *Analyze* your role:

Step 3. *Diagnose* the results of past behavior:

Step 4. *Clarify* your goals:

Step 5. *Prescribe* treatment:

Step 6. *Implement* treatment strategy:

Step 7. *Observe* consequences of treatment:

**Personal Practice
Learning Activities**

Step 8. *Evaluate* results:

Step 9. *Maintain* or *Modify* plan:

Step 10. *Review* and/or *Repeat:*

D. Situation 4 (Describe a problem with a friend)

Step 1. *Identify* the problem:

Step 2. *Analyze* your role:

Step 3. *Diagnose* the results of past behavior:

Step 4. *Clarify* your goals:

**Personal Practice
Learning Activities**

Step 5.   *Prescribe* treatment:

Step 6.   *Implement* treatment strategy:

Step 7.   *Observe* consequences of treatment:

Step 8.   *Evaluate* results:

Step 9.   *Maintain* or *Modify* plan:

Step 10.   *Review* and/or *Repeat:*

Personal Practice Answers to Activities 2 and 3.
Learning Activities

---

1. Answers to Activity 2:

    D-1   B-3   E-5
    F-2   A-4   C-6

2. Feeling words that would be appropriate in the responses to the situations described in Activity 3.

    A.   Disappointed, angry, irritated
    B.   Frustrated, helpless, lonely, relieved
    C.   Frustrated, angry, scared, annoyed, resentful, hurt
    D.   Rejected, doubtful, discouraged, down
    E.   Anger, fear, hurt
    F.   Sad, pain, fear, sorrow, dejected
    G.   Frustrated, irritated, mad, angry, hostile
    H.   Afraid, scared, helpless, lost
    I.   Frustrated, insecure, hostile, mad
    J.   Surprised, pleased, appreciative

Post-Test   As concisely as possible, answer each of the following questions without referring to your book or other material. When finished, refer to the Chapter V post-test answer key.

---

1. What is the most important phase in developing a positive language of acceptance?

2. Compare the accepting to the unaccepting medical assistant.

3. Define respect.

4. A medical assistant who expresses her honest feeling in an appropriate and constructive manner in order to facilitate a positive relationship would be demonstrating which of the eight essential ingredients?

5. Which essential ingredient best describes a medical assistant with the ability to share and expose her own feelings, attitudes, and experiences with other people?

6. Which essential ingredient requires that most delicacy to use?

7. Define immediacy.

Post-Test

---

8. Explain the skill of paraphrasing in the communication process.

9. Why is perception-checking an important listening sub-skill?

10. Define assertiveness.

11. When do problems or conflicts occur between individuals?

12. In addition to problem-solving, how can the ten-step model be used?

13. List the eight essential ingredients which correlate with effective human relations.

14. List five positive skills used to facilitate an Effective Communication System.

**Post-Test
Answer Key**

Compare your answers to the post-test questions to the correct answers given in the following key. While your response to each question need not correspond exactly with the words used in the answers below, the meanings must be similar in order for your response to be considered correct.

If you answer eleven of the fourteen questions correctly, you will have demonstrated a satisfactory understanding of the material in Chapter V and should proceed to the Personal Practice Learning Activities if you have not completed them or to Chapter VI if you have. If you answer fewer than eleven questions correctly, you should restudy the appropriate sections of Chapter V before proceeding with the Activities or Chapter VI.

---

1. The achievement of self-awareness.

2. The accepting medical assistant addresses herself to the individual's situation. The unaccepting medical assistant judges the individual's character and personality.

3. Respect may be defined as the ability to communicate a sincere belief in the worth and dignity of every individual as a unique human being. Respect also communicates the belief that a person can make her own decisions and decide what to do or not do based on her own interests, abilities and frame of reference.

4. Genuineness.

5. Self-disclosure.

6. Confrontation.

7. Immediately is the ability to deal with what is going on right now. Immediacy is dealing with your reactions and feelings toward the patient, physician, or colleague with regard to what is happening at the moment.

8. Paraphrasing is restating the other person's message in your own words so that each person has an opportunity to deal with any misunderstandings.

9. Perception checking gives the listener an opportunity to verify her perception of what is being said, thereby avoiding misunderstandings and hurt feelings.

10. Assertiveness is expressing yourself in such a manner that your needs, wants, thoughts, feelings and desires are known to another person.

11. Problems or conflicts usually occur when the behavior of one person interferes with what another person wants or needs to do or when two people do not believe or value the same things at the same time.

**Post-Test
Answer Key**

---

12. The ten-step model may also be used to gather and assess the necessary data to make an intelligent decision.

13. The eight essential ingredients which correlate with effective human relations:
    1) Empathy
    2) Respect
    3) Genuineness
    4) Concreteness
    5) Self-disclosure
    6) Confrontation
    7) Immediacy
    8) Potency

14. Five positive skills used to facilitate an effective communication system:
    1) Silence
    2) Open-ended acknowledgment
    3) Listening
    4) Feedback
    5) Assertiveness

Related readings

---

1. Carkhuff R. *The Art of Problem Solving.* Amherst, Mass: Human Resources Development Press Inc; 1973.

2. Ellis A, Harper R. *A Guide to Successful Marriage.* North Hollywood, Calif: Wilshire Book Co; 1971.

3. Fromm E. *The Art of Loving.* New York, NY: Harper & Row; 1956.

4. Johnson D, Johnson F. *Joining Together.* Englewood Cliffs, NJ: Prentice-Hall Inc; 1975.

5. Maltz M. *Psycho-Cybernetics.* Englewood Cliffs, NJ: Prentice-Hall Inc; 1960.

6. Peale N. *The Power of Positive Thinking.* Englewood Cliffs, NJ: Prentice-Hall Inc; 1952.

7. Rogers C. *Becoming Partners.* New York, NY: Delacorte Press; 1972.

8. Rogers C. *On Becoming a Person.* Boston, Mass: Houghton Mifflin Co; 1961.

9. Satir V. *Peoplemaking.* Palo Alto, Calif: Science and Behavior Books Inc; 1972.

10. Small J. *Becoming Naturally Therapeutic.* Austin, Tex: The Texas Commission on Alcoholism; 1974.

Additional readings

Birndman R, Kirscher R. *Dealing With People You Can't Stand.* New York, NY: McGraw-Hill, Inc; 1994.

Cleland J. *Putting First What Matters Most.* New York, NY: New American Library, Division of Penguin Putnam, Inc; 2001.

Fisher R, Brown S. *Getting Together: Building Relationships As We Negotiate.* New York, NY: Penguin Books; 1988.

Ringer R. *Getting What You Want: The 7 Principles of Rational Living.* New York, NY: G.P. Putnam's Sons; 2000.

Ziglar Z. *See You at the Top.* Gretna, La: Pelican Publishing Company Inc; 1987.

Chapter VI:

Preventive medicine

**Guidelines for
Group Study**

---

1. From the book:

    A. Review the chapter objectives and competency check questions.
    B. Discuss the concept of preventive medicine and its use in the human relations field.
    C. Discuss office management.
    D. Discuss personnel management.
    E. Discuss the supervisory process.

2. From the workbook:
    A. The case studies may be used in several ways or combinations thereof:
        1) The cases can be completed by each person prior to class, with small groups formed during class to discuss members' responses and the suggested answers.
        2) They can be completed during class, provided there is enough time to discuss the results.
        3) The cases can be role-played and discussed by group members. It is suggested that at least 2 or 3 of the situations be role-played.

    B. The group may prefer to identify, role-play, and discuss a common problem not covered in one of the case studies presented in the workbook.

Pretest   In the space provided answer concisely each of the following questions. The answer key follows the pretest.

---

1. List four human relationship skills often used to enhance individual worth and dignity.

2. Briefly explain the advantages of a job description.

3. List the two personnel management concepts that must be considered by the health care delivery team.

4. Describe the concept of personal and professional growth and development.

5. List the five steps used in the supervisory process model.

6. The supervisory process model can be used for what purposes?

**Pretest
Answer Key**

Compare your pretest responses to the correct answers stated in the following key. If you answer five of the six questions correctly, proceed to the Personal Practice Learning Activities, as you have successfully challenged the content of this chapter. If fewer than five of your answers are correct, you should study the material in Chapter VI of the book.

Your answers need not correspond exactly to the answers in the key, but the meanings of the two responses must be similar in order for your answer to be considered correct.

---

1. 1) Complimenting an individual's proper behavior; 2) Telling people what behavior is desirable; 3) Suggesting cooperative behavior; and 4) Confronting another person when you don't agree with him. (Confrontation suggests that the other person is worthwhile and important enough for you to want to resolve any conflicts.)

2. A job description assists in preventing any misunderstandings concerning what is expected of an employee; mainly, who is to do what, with whom, where, and when.

3. 1) Evaluation, and 2) professional growth and development.

4. Work should be a meaningful and rewarding experience with opportunities for employees to grow and develop according to their abilities and to have the satisfaction of knowing they are improving. Individuals should be involved in the decision-making process regarding policies and procedures that affect their personal and professional lives, and all employees should develop an attitude and a concern for providing better health care. All members of the health care team will work hard to provide effective care when they feel a part of the team.

5. 1) Review of Job description; 2) Observation of work performance; 3) Analysis of data; 4) Supervisor-supervisee conference; 5) Internalization and critique of process.

6. Evaluation purposes and/or professional growth purposes.

**Personal Practice
Learning Activities**

The following case studies simulate interpersonal problems frequently encountered by medical assistants and will provide you with opportunities to apply what you have learned from your study of *Human Relations: Nourishment for the Medical Practice.*

Each case study begins with a description of the situation, and your first assignment (Activity A) is to respond to the message being sent in the case description. After you have selected the response that you believe most effectively responds to the message, you should check your answer with the discussion of case studies on page 121 before proceeding with Activities B and C. These two activities build on your response to Activity A, so it is important that you know the correct answer before completing B and C.

---

1. You are a new employee, and there are two other medical assistants in the office, Jane and Anne. Jane does the administrative work, and Anne's duties are primarily clinical. You were hired because of your ability to work in both clinical and administrative areas, but your specific duties have never been stipulated and none of the employees has a job description. After a patient leaves an examining room one day, Dr. Jones impatiently says to you, "Can you keep better track of the room supplies? There are no tongue depressors in this room."

    A. Which of the following is the best response?

       1) "You seem impatient, and I am confused because I don't know what my responsibilities are."

       2) 'I didn't realize that keeping the examining rooms supplied was my responsibility."

       3) "Isn't keeping the examining rooms supplied Anne's responsibility?"

       4) "I'll take care of the matter, Dr. Jones, and can assure you that it won't happen again."

    B. What would you do then?

    C. What would the probable result of this interaction be?

Personal Practice
Learning Activities

---

2. An out-of-town patient, Mrs. Smith, habitually comes to see the physician without an appointment. One day she drops in around 2:30 PM for a routine check-up. The physician is not only booked solid for the rest of the day but also unusually behind schedule because of an emergency, and there are many patients waiting in the reception room. You explain to Mrs. Smith that the physician simply will not be able to see her and offer to make an appointment for the next week. The physician overhears your conversation and summons you to his office to say, "Mrs. Smith has driven so far … I think you should work her in as soon as possible."

    A. You would tell that physician that:

        1) Mrs. Smith abuses the fact that she is from out of town and that many patients drive just as far.

        2) He is being just too kind-hearted in this situation.

        3) His interfering in your decisions makes it difficult for you to deal with patients, and in this case you cannot reverse your decision without losing the patient's respect.

        4) You recognize his concern for keeping Mrs. Smith happy, but point out that there are many patients with appointments who are waiting to see him.

    B. How would you prevent recurrences of this type of problem with the physician?

    C. What do you think the result of your interaction with the physician would be?

**Personal Practice
Learning Activities**

---

3. You work for an internist, Dr. Smith. One afternoon an unaccompanied elderly lady comes into your office on her way to another physician who has an office in the same building, six floors up and at the opposite end. The lady is ashen-faced, seems to be in acute pain, and says, "Help me. My stomach hurts so bad!"

    A. Which of the following is the best response?

        1) "Oh, you poor lady! Sit down and rest a minute."

        2) "The pain must be terrible. Sit here, and I'll get Dr. Smith."

        3) "Shall I call your doctor for you?"

        4) "Sit here and rest a bit ... then you can go to your own doctor."

        5) "I'm so sorry ... try not to think about the pain."

    B. What would you do next?

    C. What would you expect the result of your interaction with the lady to be?

**Personal Practice
Learning Activities**

4. Thinking that filing Medicare claims is routine office procedure, a new medical assistant takes a patient's Medicare number and tells him that another medical assistant (you) will file his claim. The patient subsequently receives an itemized statement (adequate for Medicare purposes) and Medicare form, along with instructions to complete the top portion of the form and mail it and the statement to Medicare. He angrily marches into the office, is referred to you, and says, "Doesn't anyone around here know what's going on?"

   A. Which of the following is the best response?

       1) "Don't get mad at me. You were given the wrong information."

       2) "It's really quite simple to complete the form and will take only a minute."

       3) "I'm sorry, but you'll have to complete the form and mail it yourself."

       4) "You seem pretty upset with this mix-up. Let me show you how to complete the top portion of the form."

       5) "Filing such forms is the patient's responsibility … we would have to increase our costs if we were to do it."

   B. How should you handle this patient's anger?

   C. What result would you expect your interactions to bring?

**Personal Practice
Learning Activities**

---

5. You work for Doctors Henry and Davis, who are partners in a psychiatric practice. Dr. Henry does a considerable amount of personal dictation, which you willingly transcribe and handle. Dr. Davis does not ask you to handle his personal correspondence, and one day tells you to not do Dr. Henry's during office hours. He comments, "I just don't understand anybody wanting to have personal business handled by office personnel."

A. You would say to Dr. Davis that:

1) You agree and really would prefer not having to do it.

2) It doesn't take much time, you don't object to doing it, and that you'd be glad to do his as well.

3) He seems to resent your handling Dr. Henry's personal correspondence, although you don't object to it, and that perhaps he should talk to Dr. Henry about it.

4) Dr. Henry participates in many civic-oriented activities, and that you feel you are doing your share by helping Dr. Henry do his work.

5) You feel it's a matter for you and Dr. Heney to decide.

B. How would you attempt to resolve this situation where you seem to be caught between two physicians?

C. What do you think the result of your efforts would be?

Personal Practice
Learning Activities

---

6. Office personnel are very busy and falling behind in the work, partly because one of your co-workers frequently makes personal telephone calls during office hours. After one of her phone calls, she say to you, "I just love this job. I have so much free time to talk with my friends."

    A. You would:

        1) Comment that she seems to enjoy talking with her friends, but that there is a lot of work to do and the office is falling behind.

        2) Comment that she would not have so much time to talk if she did her full share of the work and express your dissatisfaction with having to do some of hers.

        3) Say that you've been meaning to talk with her about her personal use of the office telephone.

        4) Confide that you wish you had more friends to talk with on office time, since the physician never complains about the telephone being used for personal calls.

        5) Suggest that she stop tying up the office phone with personal telephone calls.

    B. What further action would you take?

    C. What would you expect the result of your action to be?

**Personal Practice
Learning Activities**

---

7. At 3 o'clock in the afternoon, the mother-in-law of a female patient who had had surgery early that morning, calls to learn what was done and why. After you decline to answer her questions, she says, "What do you mean you can't tell me what the doctor found"?

    A. Which of the following is the best response?

        1) "I am sorry, but only the physician can give out that information."

        2) "You'll have to obtain that information from your daughter-in-law."

        3) "I sense your concern for your daughter-in-law, but I am not qualified, or permitted by professional ethics, to explain her surgery to you."

        4) "I'm not really sure what was found, but don't worry … everything will be fine."

    B. What further action, if any, should you take?

    C. What would you expect the result of you interactions with the mother-in-law to be?

Discussion of Case Studies   Compare your responses to the case study activities with the answers given below.

Remember to check your answer to Activity A within each case before proceeding to Activities B and C because these latter activities build on the correct response to A.

---

1. Activity A: Response #1 is the best because it acknowledges the feeling of both parties and attempts to identify the problem.

   Activity B: It would probably benefit you to tell the physician (using the assertive skills discussed in Chapter V) what you are presently doing and to find out specifically what he wants you to do. After his expectations of you are clarified, you will better understand your role and office responsibilities. The suggested procedures in Chapter VI for developing a job description should be helpful. (As a point of information, this problem could have been prevented if job descriptions had been prepared for each employee and reviewed with each when they were hired.)

   Activity C: The result will probably be a better understanding of what the physician expects of you. The physician will also respect you for being able to clarify the situation in a tactful way.

2. Activity A: Response #4 is the best because it acknowledges the physician's feeling first and then tactfully confronts him with the possible ill-will his decision could generate.

   Activity B: It would probably be helpful for you to share, at an appropriate time and place, your feelings of frustration with the physician. Such a sharing should lead to a clarification of his attitudes and expectations.

   Activity C: The result will probably be a mutual understanding of and agreement on how similar situations will be handled in the future.

3. Activity A: Response #2 is the best because it acknowledges the patient's feelings and then suggests remedial action. The medical assistant responding in this way indicated she is an accepting person and situation-oriented.

   Activity B: After letting the lady know you recognize her suffering, immediately seek the physician in your office. He can determine whether the lady needs immediate treatment or can be helped to her original destination.

   Activity C: The lady will either be treated by your physician or be assisted to the proper office. In either case and as a secondary benefit, she will have positive feelings about you and your office.

**Discussion of
Case Studies**

---

4. Activity A: Response #4 is the best because, again, it indicates that the medical assistant first acknowledges the man's feelings and then focuses on the situation.

   Activity B: The patient's anger should be recognized and responded to first and then the procedure explained. Immediately becoming defensive about office procedure would not resolve the problem and would probably irritate the patient even more.

   Activity C: Once the patient understands that procedure, he should feel more positive about you and your office. With guidance from you, he will probably sit down and complete the top portion of the form.

5. Activity A: Response #3 is the best because it first recognized the feelings of Dr. Davis, then states how the medical assistant feels, and finally suggests a possible remedial approach.

   Activity B: This situation is quite delicate but could be handled appropriately in one of two ways: 1) As suggested in the correct response to Activity A, you should appropriately assert yourself and tell Dr. Davis how you feel and then suggest that he discuss the situation with Dr. Henry, since he (Dr. Davis) is the person unhappy with the situation. 2) You might prefer to schedule a joint meeting with both physicians to share your frustrations and confusion about what is expected of you. Either approach should be effective if you assert yourself appropriately and use the communication skills discussed in Chapter V.

   Activity C: The result should be a clarification and understanding of your duties with regard to the personal concerns of the physicians. Negative feelings between the two physicians regarding this matter should also be eliminated.

6. Activity A: Response #1 is the best because it deals with the situation rather than the co-worker's character.

   Activity B: You should appropriately assert yourself in discussing with your co-worker your feelings about the personal telephone calls and how they affect you and the office work.

   Activity C: Your feelings should be clarified, as well as the effects of the co-worker's behavior on you. The ten-step problem-solving approach outlined in Chapter V can be used to negotiate a solution acceptable to both parties. (This problem might have been prevented if the office policy regarding personal phone calls had been made clear to all new employees at the time of hiring *and* stated in the office policy manual.)

**Discussion of
Case Studies**

---

7. Activity A: Response #3 is best because it acknowledges the woman's concern and explains why the medical assistant cannot answer her questions.

    Activity B: After responding to the mother-in-law's interest and concern, you should refer her to the physician.

    Activity C: The mother-in-law will feel that her daughter-in-law is in the hands of professional health care deliverers, and she will probably be more agreeable to following proper procedures for seeking information about the family members.

Post-Test   As concisely as possible, answer each of the following questions without referring to your book or other material. When finished, refer to the Chapter VI post-test answer key.

---

1. With regard to meeting people's needs, what is the distinguishing characteristic of a successful medical practice?

2. List four techniques or skills that can be used to tell people what they need to know in such a way that their feelings of worth and dignity are enhanced.

3. A well-written job description will clarify to an employee what is expected of her. How else can it be used?

4. List at least four topics which should be covered in a patient education brochure.

5. Why should the medical assistant in charge of scheduling appointments ask each patient in advance the reason for his visit?

6. List the two personnel management concepts of most importance to the health care team.

---

7. Contrast the medical assistant who has a "career" attitude with the medical assistant who has a "job" attitude.

8. State three qualities effective supervisors have.

9. List in their correct order the five steps of the effective supervisory process.

10. Describe how a supervisor should analyze the data collected while observing a supervisee's job performance.

**Post-Test
Answer Key**

Compare your answers to the post-test questions to the correct answers given in the following key. While your response to each question need not correspond exactly to the words used in the answers below, the meanings must be similar in order for your response to be considered correct.

If you answer eight of the ten questions correctly, you have demonstrated a satisfactory understanding of the material in Chapter VI and should proceed to the Personal Practice Learning Activities if you have not completed them. If you answer fewer than eight of the questions correctly, you should restudy the appropriate sections of Chapter VI before preceding.

One Chapter VI is completed, you will be ready for the final examination. A review of the chapter pretests and post-tests is recommended before the final examination is attempted.

---

1. The concern for meeting the needs of patients and health care team members.

2. 1) Complimenting an individual's proper behavior; 2) Telling people what behavior is desirable; 3) Suggesting cooperative behavior; and 4) Confronting another person when you don't agree with him. (Confrontation suggests that the other person is worthwhile and important enough for you to want to resolve any conflicts.)

3. For self-evaluation by the employee and performance evaluation by the employee's supervisor.

4. Among those you might have listed are: Office hours, payment and billing procedures, appointment scheduling and cancelling, hospitals used by the physician, parking information, what to do in an emergency, office procedures pertinent to your particular specialty.

5. So that an appropriate amount of time can be reserved in the office schedule. Effective scheduling enhances patient relations, as well as intra-office relationships.

6. 1) Evaluation, and 2) professional growth and development.

7. The career-minded medical assistant is interested in contributing to her profession and improving her abilities; she is often involved in continuing education programs. The job-oriented medical assistant is primarily interested in monetary returns and has little or no interest in continuing education programs or improving her job-related skills.

8. 1) The expectation that their supervisees will be successful.
    2) The ability to gain the respect, trust, and understanding of co-workers.
    3) Good listening and problem-solving skills.

9. 1) Review of job description; 2) Observation of work performance; 3) Analysis of data; 4) Supervisor-supervisee conference; 5) Internalization and critique of process.

Post-Test
Answer Key

10. The supervisor should first list all the positive aspects of the supervisee's performance. Secondly, the supervisor should consider those aspects of the supervisee's performance that seemed most difficult. Thirdly, the supervisor should consider the alternative ways the supervisee might have performed her tasks, including tasks done well, as well as those done poorly. Finally, the supervisor should plan how to present her information to the supervisee during Step 4 of the process, the Supervisor-Supervisee conference.

Related readings

1. *The Business Side of Medical Practice.* Chicago, Ill: American Medical Association; 1973.

2. Dallas R, Thompson J. *Clerical and Secretarial Systems for the Office.* Englewood Cliffs, NJ: Prentice-Hall Inc; 1975.

3. *Medical Office Forms and Procedures/A Sample Manual.* Chicago, Ill: American Association of Medical Assistants Inc; 1975.

4. Saltonstall R. *Human Relations in Administration.* New York, NY: McGraw-Hill Book Company Inc; 1959.

Additional readings

Allen D. *Getting Things Done.* New York, NY: Penguin Putnam, Inc; 2000.

Bodin M. *Using the Telephone More Effectively.* Hauppauge, NY: Barron's Educational Series, Inc; 1997.

Byham W. *Zapp: The Lightning of Empowerment.* New York, NY: Harmony Books; 1988.

Glasser W. *The Control Theory Manager.* New York, NY: Harper Collins Publishers, Inc; 1994.

Heller R. *Communicate Clearly.* New York, NY: DK Publishing, Inc; 1998.

Morgenstern J. *Organizing From The Inside Out.* New York, NY: Henry Holt & Co., LLC; 1998.

Rogak L. *Smart Guide to Managing Your Time.* New York, NY: John Wiley & Sons, Inc; 1999.

**Directions for the
Final Examination**

This section of the workbook contains the final examination for AAMA's Continuing Education course on Human Relations. Course enrollees who correctly answer 70% of the 50 questions will be awarded 45 CEUs (30 gen, 15 adm) by the American Association of Medical Assistants.

Before attempting the examination, we encourage you to review the chapter summaries and competency check questions in the book and the post-tests in your workbook. Such a review should maximize the likelihood of your earning a passing score on the examination. When you have finished your review, proceed according to the following directions.

1. The examination should be completed under examination conditions: You should be in a distraction-free room and sitting at a desk or table with adequate lighting and space for you materials. You should have at least one hour for the examination that will be free of anticipated interruptions, demands, or appointments, and you must put aside all reference material.

2. You will need a black pen.

3. Take out the answer sheet, inserted at the back of this workbook.

4. To ensure the proper recording of CEU credit, provide your name, address, and social security number on the back of the answer sheet.

5. Fill in the circle for each answer.

6. After completing this examination, please double check to make sure your name, address, and social security number are on the back of your answer sheet. Then, put it in an envelope and mail it to:

> Continuing Education Department
> American Association of Medical Assistants
> 20 N. Wacker Drive, Suite 1575
> Chicago, IL 60606

Final Examination—Form A

---

1. A medical assistant who wishes to improve her interpersonal relationships should *first:*

    a. imitate significant others who have good interpersonal relationships.
    b. achieve self-awareness.
    c. develop a positive ratio concept.
    d. develop a positive self-concept.
    e. communicate effectively.

2. Most problems and concerns of people are:

    a. financial.
    b. interpersonal.
    c. exaggerated.
    d. professional.
    e. psychosomatic.

3. The happiest and most successful people are usually those who have:

    a. a secure job.
    b. a way with other people.
    c. a professional education.
    d. financial security.
    e. good health.

4. Social learning is the learning of:

    a. customs and mores shared by many societies and cultures.
    b. principles of sociology.
    c. behaviors considered appropriate and desirable by a society.
    d. theories relevant to the study of human relationships.
    e. a society's culture and history.

5. Understanding self and others is essentially a matter of:

    a. genuineness.
    b. awareness.
    c. interest.
    d. intelligence.
    e. sincerity.

6. A work environment that will contribute the most to one's social interactions is:

    a. stimulating.
    b. secure.
    c. relaxed.
    d. challenging.
    e. fast-paced.

7. The one factor which has the most influence on behavior is:

   a. awareness.
   b. self-concept.
   c. interpersonal relationships.
   d. communication style.
   e. social development.

8. Retaining individuality while simultaneously making compromises to obtain group acceptance is known as:

   a. individualization.
   b. identification.
   c. acculturation.
   d. socialization.
   e. specialization.

9. Attempting to assume the roles, attitudes, feelings, and behaviors of another person is known as:

   a. imitation.
   b. individualization.
   c. identification.
   d. socialization.
   e. specialization.

10. The reaction a person receives from others in response to certain behavior is called:

   a. input.
   b. output.
   c. result.
   d. process.
   e. feedback.

11. In Ojemann's Behavior Equation, IPS stands for:

   a. immediate physical setting.
   b. interactions per second.
   c. immediate personal satisfaction.
   d. implied psychological satisfaction.
   e. imminent probable selection.

12. According to Maslow, which of the following needs is most rarely satisfied?

   a. Physical safety.
   b. Esteem.
   c. Respect.
   d. Self-actualization.
   e. Love.

13. Perceptual psychologists believe that an individual's behavior at any given moment is the result of:

   a. how he sees himself.
   b. his motivating forces.
   c. his childhood experiences.
   d. environmental determinants.
   e. genetic determinants.

14. According to Gordon, the person experiencing frustration:

    a. is trying to satisfy third level needs.
    b. "owns" the problem.
    c. has an "I'm not OK" attitude.
    d. has a "You're not OK" attitude.
    e. is communicating from the child ego state.

15. In Transactional Analysis, the ego state which processes information is the:

    a. little professor.
    b. adult.
    c. natural child.
    d. critical parent.
    e. nurturing parent.

16. Which of the following is the best example of a hereditary characteristic?

    a. Hair texture.
    b. Hair style.
    c. Communication style.
    d. Self-concept.
    e. Belief system.

17. The causal approach to explaining human behavior is best summed up by which of the following expressions?

    a. Perceptual psychology.
    b. Maslow's hierarchy of needs.
    c. MF + R + IPS = Behavior.
    d. Transactional analysis.
    e. Effective communications.

18. To deal effectively with weakness and liabilities, one should:

    a. concentrate on eliminating them.
    b. turn them into strengths and assets.
    c. deny they exist.
    d. accept them as obstacles.
    e. concentrate on improving strengths.

19. The successful medical assistant is likely to:

    a. be introverted.
    b. be extroverted.
    c. communicate as a "sweet talker."
    d. communicate as an "expert."
    e. see herself as needed and attractive.

20. A medical assistant believes she is an efficient office manager, but a well-respected physician tells her physician-employer that the office is inefficient. This feedback will most likely affect the medical assistant's self-concept by:

    a. strengthening her self-concept.
    b. reinforcing her self-concept.
    c. causing a conflict in her self-concept.
    d. being screened out by her self-concept.
    e. having no effect on her self-concept.

21. Proponents of TA believe that behavior can be understood by:

    a. analyzing one's dreams.
    b. investigating one's relationships with early authority figures.
    c. considering verbal exchanges between ego states.
    d. studying how one perceives himself and his situation.
    e. learning one's motivating forces.

22. With regard to psychological characteristics, the successful medical assistant:

    a. understands psychological theories.
    b. does not let her personal problems affect professional behavior.
    c. tries to satisfy her personal needs.
    d. is motivated to work by monetary compensation.
    e. is generous with those who treat her well.

23. Confronting others is a way of:

    a. starting an argument.
    b. settling a disagreement.
    c. sharing your concerns and feelings.
    d. enhancing your self-concept.
    e. getting people to do what you want.

24. The best way a medical assistant can enhance her capacity to care for other people is to:

    a. increase her medical knowledge.
    b. develop a good self-image and self-respect.
    c. study human behavior.
    d. learn to communicate offensively.
    e. become an expert problem-solver.

25. Which of the following has the most direct effect on face-to-face communications?

    a. The 4-A Formula.
    b. The Behavior Equation.
    c. Personal Resources.
    d. Environment.
    e. Hidden objectives.

26. The most common cause of unproductive communication is:

    a. negative self-image.
    b. ignorance.
    c. poor environment.
    d. poor health.
    e. insensitivity.

27. A person who becomes too wrapped up in details is probably doing so:

    a. to gain a reputation for being exceptionally thorough.
    b. out of fear she will make a mistake.
    c. because she enjoys solving problems.
    d. to strengthen her self-image.
    e. to avoid dealing with feelings and emotions.

28. Sympathizing is a barrier to effective communication when the:

    a. recipient is not effectively reassured.
    b. recipient is encouraged to dwell on her problems.
    c. 10-step approach is not implemented.
    d. problem is not identified correctly.
    e. recipient's feeling are ignored.

29. The barrier of advising implies that the recipient of the advice:

    a. can't solve her own problem.
    b. is a fence rider.
    c. communicates defensively.
    d. is not willing to take risks.
    e. is a critic.

30. An acceptable ration between positive and negative statements in the effective communication system would be:

    a. Five positive for every negative one.
    b. One positive for one negative.
    c. Three positive for two negative.
    d. Three negative for one positive.
    e. Five negative for every positive one.

31. Respect, as used in the Effective Communications System, will most often help other people:

    a. get in touch with their true feelings.
    b. deal with abstract information.
    c. accept responsibility for their own behavior.
    d. evaluate the results of their treatment-strategy.
    e. develop perception-checking skills.

32. The successful medical practice is characterized by a concern for:

    a. indigent patients.
    b. establishing a positive ratio between supervisors and supervisees.
    c. eradicating disease.
    d. meeting patient and staff needs.
    e. preventive medicine.

33. The ability to deal with what is going on at the moment is:

    a. awareness.
    b. empathy.
    c. immediacy.
    d. concreteness.
    e. potency.

34. The ability to point out discrepancies is known as:

    a. assertion.
    b. confrontation.
    c. awareness.
    d. perception checking.
    e. paraphrasing.

35. An open-ended acknowledgment is:

    a. a listening sub-skill.
    b. a way of telling another person you have heard him.
    c. often an invitation to say more.
    d. B & C of the above.
    e. A, B, and C of the above.

36. Medical Assistant "A" works in an unorganized office with three other medical assistants, one of whom is her supervisor. Medical Assistant "A" decides to develop her own job description in an effort to reduce the number of misunderstandings about who is responsible for what. Her first step is to:

    a. discuss her responsibilities with the supervisor.
    b. arrange for a performance evaluation.
    c. request a staff meeting to discuss office problems.
    d. prepare a list of tasks she performs.
    e. decide which tasks she would like to do on a regular basis.

37. The effective supervisor is respected and trusted by co-workers primarily because she:

    a. has good problem-solving skills.
    b. communicates offensively.
    c. fairly represents their interests in staff meetings.
    d. respects and trusts co-workers.
    e. all of the above.

38. The first step of the Effective Supervisory Process is:

    a. involving the team members in decision-making.
    b. observing work performance.
    c. setting reasonable objectives.
    d. writing the job description.
    e. reviewing the job description.

39. Which of the following is a distinguishing characteristic of an effective health care team?

    a. Members are self-actualized.
    b. Members are personal friends.
    c. The presence of hidden objectives.
    d. A willingness to change.
    e. The desire to cure every disease.

40. We store our most important pictures of people, places and things that help us meet our needs in our

    a. quality world.
    b. perceived world.
    c. comparing place.
    d. behavioral system.
    e. real world.

41. Choice Theory is an explanation of how the brain works as a control system.

    a. true
    b. false

42. Glasser says "external control psychology" destroys relationships.

    a. true
    b. false

43. In the past 100 years we have made gigantic progress in human relations.

    a. true
    b. false

44. When we "sharpen the saw" we are being good to ourselves.

    a. true
    b. false

45. Being proactive means to captain our own ship.

    a. true
    b. false

46. In a competitive world we must be sure our point of view is understood before we worry about another viewpoint.

    a. true
    b. false

47. The four psychological needs are freedom, fun, power and belonging.

    a. true
    b. false

48. The quality world is referred to as the all we want world.

    a. true
    b. false

49. To be synergized is to be able to solve the problem without any help.

    a. true
    b. false

50. Reality Therapy is based on the Seven Habits.

    a. true
    b. false

Final Examination—Form B

---

1. The amount of satisfaction a patient feels about the health care he receives is usually attributable to:

    a. the amount of physical discomfort suffered.
    b. whether he could afford the cost of the medical care.
    c. the nature of his interpersonal relationships with the health care providers.
    d. the effectiveness of the treatment and rate of recovery.
    e. the length and severity of his illness.

2. With regard to job performance, the American Management Association consider which of the following attributes to be the most vital?

    a. Intelligence.
    b. Ability to get along with people.
    c. Ability to make a decision.
    d. Knowledge.
    e. Creativity.

3. The most common reason people lose their jobs is:

    a. a poor attitude.
    b. lack of technical skill.
    c. failure to do the work.
    d. failure to deal successfully with people.
    e. excessive absenteeism.

4. An assumption of a behavioral control system is that:

    a. control is a matter of conditioning and experience.
    b. control is acquired through imitating significant others.
    c. communication skills can be learned.
    d. feedback is a consequence of behavior.
    e. behavior is genetically determined.

5. Which of the following usually has the greatest influence on social development?

    a. Mental resources.
    b. Education.
    c. Professional responsibility.
    d. Home environment.
    e. Personal initiative.

6. Social behavior is:

    a. cumulative.
    b. cumulative and learned.
    c. reciprocal and learned.
    d. reciprocal and cumulative.
    e. cumulative, learned, and reciprocal.

7. Socialization is society's attempt to have a person accept all of the following *except* its:

   a. values.
   b. regulations.
   c. mores.
   d. changes.
   e. behavior patterns.

8. A condition necessary for the development of social control is learning:

   a. how to individualize.
   b. how to control anger.
   c. to communicate effectively.
   d. that other people are necessary.
   e. that feedback and self-control are interdependent.

9. People who require almost constant interaction with other people can best be described as:

   a. extroverted.
   b. introverted.
   c. humanistic.
   d. asocial.
   e. antisocial.

10. In Ojemann's Behavior Equation, the "Motivating Forces" include all of the following *except:*

    a. sexual.
    b. physiological.
    c. talents.
    d. social.
    e. psychological.

11. Which of the following does Maslow consider a third level need?

    a. Shelter.
    b. Belonging.
    c. Safety.
    d. Respect.
    e. Esteem.

12. The one need that is not psychological in Glasser's Choice Theory is:

    a. belonging.
    b. power.
    c. survival.
    d. freedom.
    e. fun.

13. According to Thomas Gordon, all behavior can be classified as:

    a. effective or ineffective.
    b. productive and unproductive.
    c. acceptable or unacceptable.
    d. constructive or destructive.
    e. none of the above.

14. Smiles, praise, frowns, and criticism are examples of:

    a. rituals.
    b. games.
    c. transactions.
    d. strokes.
    e. pastimes.

15. When people say one thing and mean another, the transaction is:

    a. covert.
    b. crossed.
    c. complimentary.
    d. contrived.
    e. parallel.

16. To completely understand herself, the medical assistant must:

    a. have a positive self-concept.
    b. be sensitive to others.
    c. believe in the worth of her work.
    d. be able to share herself with another person.
    e. be an approachable person.

17. Self-concept will be promoted by all of the following *except:*

    a. learning from the mistakes of others.
    b. practicing positive communication skills.
    c. speaking and operating from the positive.
    d. developing an "I'm OK" attitude.
    e. being open and honest with self and others.

18. A sincere smile is an example of which of the following types of characteristics?

    a. Psychological.
    b. Social.
    c. Physical.
    d. Mental.
    e. Genetic.

19. The "4-A Formula" for developing social skills includes all of the following *except:*

    a. acceptance.
    b. approval.
    c. attitude.
    d. affirmation.
    e. appreciation.

20. Which of the following sequences shows the five stages of dying in their correct order as classified by Elisabeth Kübler-Ross?

    a. Depression, denial, anger, acceptance, approval.
    b. Awareness, acceptance, anger, depression, denial.
    c. Awareness, bargaining, anger, denial, depression.
    d. Denial, anger, bargaining, depression, acceptance.
    e. Denial, bargaining, anger, acceptance, depression.

21. Research suggests that a medical assistant will most likely be successful if she has a positive self-concept, believes in the worth of her work and:
    a. establishes efficient office procedures and performs competently the duties in her job description.
    b. tries to overcome her faults and communications from the adult ego state.
    c. is physically attractive and an empathetic person.
    d. values other people and focuses on their needs rather than procedures.
    e. does not bring her personal problems to the office and tries to solve problems systematically.

22. As the potential recipient of feedback, you should:
    a. avoid it.
    b. disregard it.
    c. challenge it.
    d. solicit it.
    e. minimize it.

23. Of the skills outlined in the effective communication system, which one is usually the most therapeutic?
    a. Problem-solving.
    b. Silence.
    c. Listening.
    d. Assertiveness.
    e. Feedback.

24. Interpersonal problems are usually effectively resolved when:
    a. a logical systematic approach is followed.
    b. both parties acknowledge their mistakes.
    c. both parties assert themselves appropriately.
    d. one party takes responsibility for developing the treatment strategy.
    e. the problem is identified in terms of its solution.

25. Which of the following is usually the most honest means of expression?
    a. Body language.
    b. Written communications.
    c. Spontaneous remarks.
    d. Prepared speeches.
    e. Tone of voice.

26. A person characterized as a "fence rider":
    a. seems unaware of what is happening at the moment.
    b. appears cool and confident but often feels fragile.
    c. takes advantage of other people's generosity.
    d. cannot admit having hostile feelings.
    e. can be especially detrimental in the medical office.

27. Directions to a patient in the form of a command will most likely cause him to:

   a. feel inadequate.
   b. feel misunderstood.
   c. rebel.
   d. make defensive remarks.
   e. disclose his true feelings.

28. Analyzing another person's motives for doing something can prevent effective communications because it:

   a. suggests that the recipient's feelings are unimportant.
   b. shames the recipient.
   c. implies the problem is unimportant.
   d. can be threatening to the recipient.
   e. implies the recipient is foolish.

29. The accepting medical assistant:

   a. is situation-oriented.
   b. makes value judgments about other people.
   c. focuses on a person's character.
   d. can be characterized as a "sweet talker."
   e. none of the above.

30. The first and most important step in acquiring a positive language of acceptance is:

   a. enhancing self-concept.
   b. achieving self-awareness.
   c. practicing immediacy.
   d. learning to paraphrase.
   e. identifying the problem.

31. A listening sub-skill that gives the listener an opportunity to check his understanding of what was said is:

   a. assertion.
   b. empathy.
   c. confrontation.
   d. verbalization.
   e. none of the above.

32. A medical assistant relating from an Effective Communication System is all of the following *except:*

   a. secure within herself.
   b. projecting her own attitudes on others.
   c. dealing with others here and now.
   d. able to recognize feelings in herself and others.
   e. able to respond to feelings.

33. Empathy is:

   a. analyzing what another has said.
   b. understanding another and letting him know that you do.
   c. interpreting what another is doing.
   d. rephrasing what another had said to double-check your understanding.
   e. expression your true feelings in a constructive manner.

34. Suggesting cooperative behavior to a new patient usually had the effect of:

    a. degrading his self-concept.
    b. generating a positive response.
    c. taking his mind off his illness.
    d. creating a conflict.
    e. camouflaging the proposed treatment.

35. A medical assistant characterized by a "job" attitude probably:

    a. belongs to a professional organization.
    b. is unconcerned about monetary compensation.
    c. is not studying this course.
    d. has an above-average enjoyment of the work.
    e. participates in continuing education seminars.

36. The primary purpose of a patient education brochure is to:

    a. clarify expectations of office employees.
    b. clarify expectations of the patient.
    c. prevent misunderstandings among office employees.
    d. explain federal insurance programs.
    e. explain home care procedures.

37. An especially potent quality that effective supervisors have is:

    a. ability to solicit co-operative behavior from patients.
    b. the expectation that supervisees will be successful.
    c. a positive self-concept.
    d. ability to communicate with physicians and supervisees.
    e. none of the above.

38. In addition to evaluating job performance, the effective supervisor helps supervisees:

    a. solve personal problems.
    b. grow professionally.
    c. complete their duties in a timely manner.
    d. communicate with patients and physicians.
    e. satisfy their personal needs.

39. The following component is not a part of total behavior.

    a. doing.
    b. thinking.
    c. feeling.
    d. loving.
    e. physiology.

40. The way we see our world is referred to as a

    a. synergy.
    b. thought.
    c. paradigm.
    d. truth.
    e. action.

41. Choice Theory suggests we can control anything in our lives.

    a. true
    b. false

42. Glasser says most of the misery in the world is a result of unsatisfying personal relationships.

    a. true
    b. false

43. The love and belonging need refers to reproducing.

    a. true
    b. false

44. Covey says we should begin a project with the beginning.

    a. true
    b. false

45. Putting first things first is all about commitment.

    a. true
    b. false

46. When we think win-win we are looking to treat others with respect and dignity.

    a. true
    b. false

47. The four components of total behavior are actions, thoughts, emotions and physiology.

    a. true
    b. false

48. The perceived world is referred to as the all we have world.

    a. true
    b. false

49. Doing continuing education courses offered by your professional association is a good way to sharpen the saw.

    a. true
    b. false

50. The core of Reality Therapy is to help someone evaluate the effectiveness of their present behavior.

    a. true
    b. false